Consumer's Guide to Psychiatric Drugs

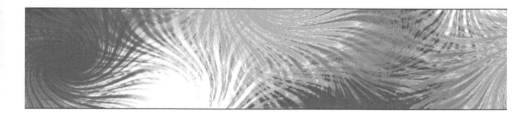

John D. Preston, Psy. D.
John H. O'Neal, M.D.
Mary C. Talaga, R.Ph., M.A.

New Harbinger Publications

Publisher's Note

This publication is designed to provide accurate and authoritative information in regard to the subject matter covered. It is sold with the understanding that the publisher is not engaged in rendering psychological, financial, legal, or other professional services. If expert assistance or counseling is needed, the services of a competent professional should be sought.

Distributed in the U.S.A. by Publishers Group West; in Canada by Raincoast Books; in Great Britain by Airlift Book Company, Ltd.; in South Africa by Real Books, Ltd.; in Australia by Boobook; and in New Zealand by Tandem Press.

Cover design by Lightbourne Images © 1997.
Edited by Kayla Sussell.
Text design by Tracy Marie Powell.

Library of Congress Catalog Card Number: 97-75482.
ISBN 1-57224-111-X Paperback.

Printed in the United States of America on recycled paper.

New Harbinger Publications' Website address: www.newharbinger.com.

First printing

To my patients, who have been my best teachers. May this book assist others, who, like them, seek help for emotional suffering.

John H. O'Neal, M.D.

To my sons, Kevin and John . . . you fill my life with joy and wonder.

Mary C. Talaga, R.Ph., M.A.

And to the memory of Carl Sagan, researcher and teacher par excellence, who believed that people from all walks of life can benefit from a knowledge of science.

John. D. Preston, Psy.D.

Contents

Acknowledgments   vii

Introduction   1

PART I Overview   5

1   Psychiatric Medication: 7
    An Historical Perspective

2   Seeking Treatment   19

3   Emotions and the Brain   25

4   Managing Your Medications   37

5   Depression   49

6   Bipolar Disorders   81

7   Anxiety Disorders   101

8   Psychotic Disorders   117

9   Miscellaneous Disorders   129
    • Sleep Disorders • Attention Deficit Disorder
    • Eating Disorders • Borderline Personality
    Disorders • Post-Traumatic Stress Disorder
    • Aggression • Dementia

10   **Medication During Pregnancy, Childhood,**   143
      Adolescence, and Old Age

11   **Nonpharmaceutical Approaches**   153

PART II   Guide to Psychiatric Drugs   161

Directory of Brand Names   163

The Guide to Psychiatric Drugs   166

References   317

Recommended Reading   323

Resources   327

Index   329

Many thanks to our publisher, Dr. Matthew McKay, and to our superb editor, Kayla Sussell, for helping our ideas to take form. Thank you to Michelle Riekstins for your help with manuscript preparation; well done, as usual.

Thanks to our family and friends, with deep appreciation for their patience and encouragement throughout this project.

Finally, special thanks to our readers. We are privileged to share in your journey toward health and happiness.

Introduction

Chances are good that because you are reading this book, either you or a family member has begun or is considering medical treatment for an emotional or psychiatric disorder. Our intention is to present a lot of practical, useful information in the hope of answering many of the questions that you may have about psychiatric treatment. We believe very strongly that everyone has a legitimate right to acquire important information about treatment and treatment options.

In the past, it was common practice for people to be examined by a doctor, given a prescription for a certain medication, told how to take it, and sent on their way. The arrangement was one of "powerful doctor" and "passive patient." As a result, many, if not most, patients felt inhibited about asking questions regarding their treatment. Fortunately, times have changed, and in our view, it is not only alright for people to inquire about their treatments, it actually makes sense for them to become informed consumers. Accurate information is not only your right, it can enhance treatment outcome and increase the likelihood of treatment success.

It is important for anyone receiving psychiatric medication treatment to know at the very least the following treatment-related information:

- What is the diagnosis?
- What are the recommended treatments for this disorder?

- If psychiatric medications are recommended:
  1. Are the recommended medications standard and well established treatments?
  2. Are the particular medications addictive?
  3. What can you expect from the medical treatment? This should include the following: (a) What are the common side effects? (b) Are any of the side effects dangerous? (c) How long must you wait to notice the positive benefits of the medication? (d) Are there any potential drug-drug interaction problems? (That is, is it dangerous to take this medication along with other prescription or over-the-counter drugs?) (e) Can you drink alcohol while taking this medication?
  4. Assuming that the medication is effective for you, how long will you have to take it?
  5. Are there any dangers in taking this medication for an extended period of time?
- Is psychotherapy recommended in addition to medication?

Of course, there may be many additional questions that will be important to address, and we encourage each of you to assert your right to inquire about any aspect of your treatment.

Possibly as much as 75 percent of all prescriptions for psychiatric medications are written by primary care and family practice doctors. And, as you well know, a typical office visit with a doctor is brief. It may be difficult if not impossible to ask all of your questions during such a brief visit. Also, if you are like most of us, a number of questions may come to your mind after your visit to the doctor, or in the days that follow. It is our hope that this book will address those questions and concerns.

The Spectrum: From Having a Bad Day to Having a Nervous Breakdown

In the chapters that follow we will be writing about a number of very common emotional and psychiatric problems. Some of these disorders are very serious but they are fairly rare (e.g., schizophrenia). Many, however, are very common; especially depression and anxiety disorders. It is important to understand that among these disorders there is a great deal of variability with regard to severity. Most of us experience occasional times of mild depression or anxiety. These times may last only a day or two, or they may be present for longer periods, causing discomfort, but not debilitation. However, it must also be understood that some anxiety and depressive disorders can become extremely severe.

At the severe end of the spectrum, anxiety and depressive disorders can become all-consuming. These illnesses can completely ruin a person's life. Not only is there great personal, emotional suffering, but there also can be a collapse into a sort of paralysis and a total inability to function. This may take the form of fearfulness that is so intense the person cannot leave home or be left alone . . . depression so engulfing that the person is literally bedridden. Depression can cause such an extreme disorganization of thinking extreme that the individual is convinced he or she is going crazy.

Certainly, a number of people can and do experience serious, chronic psychotic illnesses, although the percentage of such disorders in the general population is only about one percent. A much higher percentage of people go through very serious bouts of anxiety and depression that result in serious dysfunction. At the extreme end of this spectrum, these emotional disorders are what some of us grew up calling a "nervous" or "mental breakdown." Furthermore, these disorders can and do happen to many people who have gone through much of their lives functioning well. In fact, such grave versions of these kinds of psychiatric reactions can, under certain circumstances, strike otherwise mentally healthy individuals.

The good news is that current treatments for psychiatric disorders have a well-established record of effectiveness. The bad news is that many people suffer and never seek treatment. What is critical to understand is that emotional and psychiatric problems are very common, that most problems can be treated successfully, and that someone suffering from such a problem can take action by seeking treatment.

How to Use This Book

This book is divided into two parts. Part I consists of chapters 1 through 11, which discuss psychiatric diagnoses and specifics of medication treatment. Part II comprises a compendium of psychiatric medications providing detailed information on all specific medications. The first four chapters address a number of particular issues to help you learn more about the use of psychiatric medications. Many of our clients routinely ask about specific issues that relate to psychiatric diagnosis, the biology of emotional illnesses, and how medications work. Thus, we have attempted to speak to many of these issues in the first four chapters. What follows are chapters devoted specifically to groups of psychiatric disorders (depression, anxiety disorders, etc.). In each of these chapters we provide a great deal of specific information about treatment, including the following:

- Signs and symptoms
- How the diagnosis is made
- The role of a medical evaluation in diagnosis
- Theories about the biology of the disorder (to help explain how medications appear to work)
- Specifics of medical treatment, for example: (1) standard medical treatments; (2) details regarding treatment (e.g., recommended doses, what to expect, common side effects, etc.); (3) precautions; (4) treatment options when first-line treatments are ineffective
- Frequently recommended nonmedical treatments (e.g., types of psychotherapy)

Self-help references (books and support groups) can be found at the back of the book.

As is the case in all areas of medicine, there are a number of generally accepted, standard treatments for any particular disorder/disease. Rarely is only one approach or one medication the treatment of choice. This is certainly the case in the treatment of psychiatric disorders. Thus, this book presents the major points regarding standard psychiatric treatment for each particular disorder.

Treatment decisions will be influenced by a number of unique factors (i.e., particular symptoms, age, medical status, and so forth) and may vary from person to person. We provide general information about all the available treatments because we strongly believe that all people have the right to know as much as possible about their disorder and its treatment. However, be advised that particular treatment decisions will be unique for each individual.

Although we recommend that you read chapter 1 for some background, it is also fine to skip ahead and turn to the particular chapter that is relevant to your current concerns.

PART I

Overview

Psychiatric Medication: An Historical Perspective

Psychological Disorders Are Very Common

Since the beginning of recorded history it has been obvious that human beings are subject to a host of emotional pains. Some of these are mild, temporary, and simply annoying, while others are prolonged and a source of agony and disability. In a recent, extremely thorough, study carried out by the National Institute of Mental Health it was discovered that 48 percent of all adults in the United States will have, at least once in their lifetimes, a diagnosable psychiatric disorder. This may seem like a surprisingly large percentage, yet it appears to be quite accurate (see table 1.1).

Table 1.1
Prevalence of Psychiatric
Disorders in The United States*

Disorder	Per Year	Lifetime Prevalence
Mood disorders	11%	19%
Anxiety disorders	17%	25%

Substance abuse	11%	26%
Psychotic disorders	1%	1%

- Multiple disorders: Many individuals will have two or more disorders at the same time (e.g., depression and alcohol abuse). This is referred to as co-morbidity or co-occurrence.

- Lifetime prevalence: having any psychiatric disorder: 48%.

- Only 25% of those affected receive any form of treatment.

Negative Stigma

Despite a growing awareness and acceptance of the reality of psychological disorders, there still exists a good deal of negative stigma around psychiatric problems. In our society, emotional and psychological problems continue to be a source of shame for many people and, as a result, many of those living through difficult times are likely to keep their psychological pain private, sharing their personal feelings with no one except their closest relatives. What has become abundantly clear, however, is that the vast majority of human beings are affected by stressful and painful life events, and that many of us experience a sufficient amount of distress for this to be correctly seen as a type of psychiatric disorder.

Part of the negative stigma associated with psychological disorders frequently comes from misconceptions and inaccurate facts regarding mental and emotional illnesses. One misconception is the common notion that if you are mentally ill, weakness of character or intellect is implied. Two cases in particular underscore how far this idea is from the truth. Both Winston Churchill and Abraham Lincoln suffered from bouts of severe, clinical depression. Yet no one would question that these men were intellectually gifted, had strength of character, and were able to exert enormous influence over the histories of their nations and the lives of countless people.

Psychiatric disorders can and certainly do have a marked impact on human beings. In the midst of emotional illnesses not only do people experience overwhelming anguish, but these disorders also significantly interfere with basic functioning. Severe emotional disorders can, at least temporarily, adversely transform otherwise

---

* Does not include minor adjustment or stress disorders. Note some individuals have more than one disorder at a time (Kessler et al. 1994).

normally capable people. Many people suffering from these disorders find it very difficult to function in their day-to-day lives as productive employees, nurturing parents, and loving husbands or wives.

New Approaches to Age-Old Problems

In the early part of the twentieth century, two important events changed attitudes about psychiatric treatment and the entire landscape of mental illness and emotional suffering. The first event was a shift toward more humane treatment for people with mental illnesses. Prior to this time, those afflicted with serious psychiatric disorders were often subject to horrific "treatments" (for example, prolonged confinement in asylums). Some patients were continuously restrained in straitjackets and, in a sense, were treated more like criminals than sick people. The twentieth century has seen an increased understanding of emotional disorders as either an extension of normal human emotional responses to difficult life circumstances, or as a type of illness deserving treatment (not punishment, blame, or shame).

The second event that helped to change attitudes about emotional illnesses was the development of the first truly effective psychological treatment: psychotherapy, or as it is sometimes called, "talk therapy."

Psychological Treatment

The psychological approach to treating emotional problems was ushered in by the work of Sigmund Freud, and it has been expanded and modified in a number of ways over one-hundred years. Since the 1970s, hundreds of published research studies have demonstrated that, in general, psychotherapy is an effective treatment for a number of emotional and psychiatric disorders.

Also, the past two decades have seen the development of specific psychological therapies designed to treat specific types of disorders (e.g., cognitive therapy for the treatment of depression). Psychotherapy is often the treatment of choice for many psychological problems. There are, however, some types of psychiatric disorders for which it has demonstrated only limited success. This is especially true in the treatment of the more severe mental illnesses.

The Discovery of Psychiatric Medications

In the mid-1950s the first effective medications for treating very severe mental illnesses, such as schizophrenia and manic-depressive illness, were developed. They were hailed as godsends because, at that time, there was no other form of therapy for the more severe forms of mental illness than psychotherapy (talk therapy), and that often didn't work.

The early psychiatric medications had their problems, however; many came with a large variety of unwanted side effects and, especially in the early years, the drugs often were subject to overuse or misuse. The medications helped many patients, but they were also responsible for some disasters, especially when some patients were treated inappropriately.

During the nearly five decades since their inception, psychiatric medications have undergone significant changes. The development of new medical and scientific technologies has provided researchers with a much clearer understanding of the functioning of the brain and the biology of mental illness. Newer, safer, and more effective medications have been developed. A great deal of information has been acquired about how to prescribe treatments appropriately and how to avoid or minimize problems with side effects. Recently, new vistas have opened regarding the use of psychiatric medications for what are considered to be the less severe emotional disorders.

Common Concerns about Psychiatric Medication Treatment

The following sections describe some of the realities of psychiatric medication that initially led to hostile responses to drug treatment for emotional disorders.

Bad Press for Drug Treatment

If there was an unknown disorder that caused intense suffering for months or even years, that caused families to split up and sufferers to fail at school or lose their jobs, that interfered with health and produced prolonged spells of hopelessness, which sometimes drove people to suicide, and, finally, treatments were discovered to cure this disorder—those treatments would be heralded as miraculous. Yet when we look at the history of the development and use of psychiatric drugs for treating mental and emotional disorders (which produce all of the real-life consequences just described), the public's opinion and the media's attention often have been anything but positive. How come? There are two very good reasons that psychiatric medication treatment has been subject to such great scrutiny and such a lot of negative press.

The Chemical "Straitjacket"

The first reason psychiatric drugs received such bad press has to do with the realities of psychiatric medication treatment (especially as it was conducted during the '50s and '60s). At that time there were a great many well publicized cases in which psychiatric patients received grossly inappropriate treatment with the then-new psychiatric drugs. The most common abuse was the use of excessively high doses of tranquilizing medications, mainly to impose behavioral controls on agitated or troublesome patients. This took place primarily in state mental hospitals.

Typically, the medications were the early versions of antipsychotic drugs. These were helpful in reducing psychotic symptoms (such as hallucinations), but they were notoriously loaded with unpleasant side effects. When used in extremely high doses they did achieve behavioral control, but often at great cost in human terms. Many patients frequently were oversedated and seemed like "zombies." It was at this time that the term "chemical straitjacket" came into use.

This was also a time of great social change where free speech, personal freedom, racial equality, and civil rights became paramount values. The whole idea of restraining human beings with drugs (often completely against their will) sounded suspiciously Orwellian, and provoked outcries of protest. Although the use of psychiatric drugs did result in significantly more people being released from state hospitals, the necessity of ongoing chemical restraint caused many to question whether the newly released patients were really better off. Many opponents of psychiatric medication treatment (most notably, Dr. Thomas Szaaz) argued that the new drugs were robbing people of their humanity and individuality. The question was raised: Were these new discoveries truly medical breakthroughs, or were they simply a new technology for mind control?

Mothers' Little Helpers

The second reason that psychiatric medication treatment was not well received also began to emerge in the sixties when the minor tranquilizers (such as Miltown, Librium, and Valium) were prescribed widely by family practice doctors. They were dispensed as treatment for a variety of maladies such as frayed nerves, insomnia, tearfulness, and generalized sadness or disappointment with life. These drugs became known as "Mother's Little Helpers" (popularized as such in the Rolling Stones' song). They were seen as a panacea for many of life's woes—"Just swallow one or two and mellow out." Eventually, the darker side of using mothers' little helpers became apparent.

Questions were raised: Could it be that the main effect of the tranquilizers, so prescribed, was to induce a state of relative, albeit temporary, oblivion for unhappy housewives? Might this state of drug-induced numbness be a way to keep women in their place and perpetuate the status quo of the male-dominated society? If women were sufficiently anesthetized, maybe they would either not notice or find a way to tolerate an obnoxious or dissatisfying lifestyle (e.g., spousal abuse, or passive subservience). In a broader, less politicized, scheme, the question is reframed as: Do psychiatric medications inhibit autonomy? Do they somehow conceal or hide one's inner, truer self?

Psychiatric Medication Treatment and the Issue of Autonomy

Does psychiatric medication inhibit autonomy? This question raises an important issue in Western culture where individual freedom and expression are so highly valued. It is an even more important question in the context of the feminist movement, which has aimed to empower women and to combat the social forces that otherwise keep women powerless or in servitude. These are legitimate issues with far-reaching consequences.

Jill's Case

Jill was a thirty-four-year-old woman; a housewife, and the mother of two children. Her early life had been like that of many people growing up in a small town in America. She came from a stable and loving family, had the ordinary experiences of youth, and could not recall any remarkably traumatic or stressful times while growing up. After high school she attended a nearby college. Upon graduation, she found a job with an insurance company. In the years that followed, she married and had children. She had a good life and was grateful for it. At the age of twenty-four it would have seemed impossible to her that ten years later she would be completely unable to leave her home or to be alone for more than a few minutes without experiencing overwhelming surges of panic. She would have been incapable of imagining that in a decade she would be contemplating suicide on a daily basis.

Jill had her first panic attack at the age of thirty. She experienced a sudden eruption of intense, overwhelming fear . . . her heart began to race and she felt short of breath and dizzy. She became convinced that she was going to die at any moment. This episode came on for no apparent reason; she was sitting in a coffee shop with a friend, when panic engulfed her.

In the following week she had four additional attacks, each identical to the first. She and her husband were both sure that she had some kind of serious medical problem. Later that week she was admitted to the emergency room complaining of chest pains and an overwhelming sense of dread and panic. After a careful evaluation, she was told that she was having an anxiety attack, given reassurance that there was nothing medically wrong with her, and sent home. But she did not feel reassured at all. She was still frightened out of her wits.

During the next three months as the attacks continued, Jill did what many other people in her situation do . . . she began to develop intense fears about leaving her home. She had had attacks there too, but it was familiar turf and she felt safer there. She did not get further medical attention, but did start to drink a lot of alcohol in an attempt to quell her nerves. In five short months her life was transformed. She quit her job, stopped attending social functions, and became less and less involved in the lives of her two kids. Her life was focused on the ever-present dread, "When will the next attack occur?"

After four years of this, she was an emotional cripple. She was unable and unwilling to leave her house. And, to her great shame, her husband had to hire a "baby-sitter" to be with her during the day because she could not bear to be alone. Jill's life had been completely transformed. She was chronically depressed and lived in constant fear about the next anxiety attack.

Jill's story is not uncommon. She was suffering from severe panic disorder, and it ruined her life. This kind of psychiatric disorder rarely goes away without treatment. Fortunately for Jill, she finally did seek psychiatric treatment. At a point of utter desperation, she made an appointment with a therapist. After a careful evaluation she was told that she was suffering from a treatable emotional illness, and the therapist recommended a combined approach that included psychiatric medications (in her case, an antidepressant) and a type of psychotherapy called cognitive-behavior therapy. This combined approach—medications and cognitive-behavioral therapy—is a standard, very effective treatment for panic disorder. Initially, Jill was reluctant to take medications, so it was important for the therapist to spend a good deal of time answering her questions about the medication. It was also crucial for her to know that the choice of whether to try medication was entirely hers. On her second visit to the therapist she decided to follow the recommendation and tried the medication.

After two months of treatment, she was radically different. The panic attacks stopped and for the first time in years she was able to re-enter her normal life . . . able to attend school functions with her children . . . to visit her parents . . . and to go out on a "date" with her husband. Eventually, Jill returned to work and pursued the career that she had loved. She had found herself and was able to reclaim her life.

Although it is true that initially there were far too many instances in which psychiatric medications were misused to stifle "aliveness," free choice, and autonomy, in Jill's case we see just the opposite. The medication helped to free her from an engulfing disorder and enabled her to reclaim her true self.

These days, when people are treated with modern psychiatric medication, one of the most common remarks therapists hear once the medications begin to take effect is, "I am beginning to feel like myself again." This is a very important point to emphasize. Although some medications do have unpleasant side effects, and some misuse of these drugs certainly continues, the goal of appropriate psychiatric treatment is twofold: (1) to reduce human suffering and (2) to promote the development and expression of autonomy. This is a far cry from the chemical straitjackets of the mental hospitals' back wards in the 1950s.

Drug Addiction

Prior to the mid-1950s, some drugs were being used in psychiatry. Most, however, were very ineffective, and many were recognized as potentially addictive and dangerous. Such drugs included alcohol, marijuana, bromides, barbiturates, and amphetamines. Cultural awareness of escalating drug abuse in the 1960s sensitized the medical profession as well as the general public to the hazards of drug addiction. As the poet Robert Bly noted, "The drugged state is the fastest growing state in the union."

Unfortunately, some of the newer drugs developed in the mid-50s and early '60s included tranquilizers, which many individuals found to be habit-forming. Increasingly, in those years, when psychiatric drugs were portrayed in the media, they were discussed as if they were all the same . . . they all had terrible side effects . . . they all were habit-forming, . . . and they all were being used to achieve behavioral control. This journalistic error continues, to some degree, to this day.

Medications and the Media

Research studies and clinical experience certainly influence therapists' prescribing practices. However, in recent years the media has also had a profound effect on public opinion and ultimately on medical practice. In the late 1980s, negative media attention was focused on the drug Ritalin, a widely prescribed stimulant medication used to treat hyperactivity and attention deficit disorder. Psychiatrist Andrew Brotman, summarizing the work of Safer and Krager (1992) states, "The media attack was lead by major national television talk show hosts and in the opinion of the authors, allowed anecdotal and unsubstantiated allegations concerning Ritalin to be aired. There were also over twenty lawsuits initiated throughout the country, most by a lawyer linked to the Church of Scientology" (Brotman 1992).

In their study, conducted in Baltimore County, Maryland, of the effects of the negative media and litigation blitz Safer and Krager found that the use of Ritalin had dropped significantly. In the two-year period during and just following the negative media attention, there was a 40 percent decrease in the number of prescriptions prescribed for Ritalin. (The use of Ritalin had increased fivefold during the prior six-year period.)

Furthermore, this decrease occurred at a time when research on Attention Deficit Disorder (ADD) and stimulant treatment continued to strongly support the safety and effectiveness of such medication. The authors state that 36 percent of the children who discontinued Ritalin use experienced major academic maladjustments (such as failing grades or being suspended) and an additional 47 percent who discontinued treatment encountered mild to moderate academic problems. While Ritalin use decreased, there was a significant (fourfold) *increase* in the prescription of tricyclic antidepressants among hyperactive children. Apparently, physicians discontinued Ritalin and then prescribed antidepressants. It is important to note that tricyclic antidepressants, although often used to treat ADD, tend to have more troublesome side effects than Ritalin, and have been implicated in six reports of cardiac deaths in children. Brotman concludes, "When there are reports in the media that lead to stigmatization of a certain drug ... there tends to be a move to other medications which have less notoriety, even if they may, in fact, be more problematic" (1992.)

More recently, following wide acclaim as a new "breakthrough drug for depression" (Cowley et al. 1990) Prozac came under attack by consumer groups and, again, by the Church of Scientology. The negative attention was sparked by a single article (Teicher et al. 1990) documenting the emergence or reemergence of suicidal ideas in six patients who had been treated with Prozac. The six patients had been diagnosed as suffering from severe depression, and in no case was there an actual suicide attempt following the onset of treatment with Prozac. But suddenly Prozac was thrust into a very unfavorable light and was the next drug in line to find itself the topic of television talk shows.

Subsequent studies have failed to find any evidence that Prozac is more likely to be associated with suicidal feelings than with any other antidepressant (Fava and Rosenbaum 1991; Beasley and Dornseif 1991). In fact, in one study the incidence of suicidal ideas was greater in patients treated with placebos or tricyclic antidepressants than in those who were treated with Prozac (Beasley and Dornseif 1991).

The Church of Scientology attempted to convince the Federal Drug Administration (FDA) to remove Prozac from the market. The FDA ruled against taking that action however, because there was no scientific evidence to support the claims made by the Church of Scientology (Burton 1991).

All medications produce some side effects. Reports of serious side effects, even if seen very infrequently, must be taken seriously and investigated systematically. There certainly is a place for skepticism and scrutiny. However, it is also important to consider the negative effect of unsubstantiated reports in the press. For example, the risk of Prozac-induced suicide appears to be extremely low, while at the same time, the suicide rate in untreated major depression is reported to be between 12 and 15 percent (Hamilton 1989, 897). Clearly, failure to treat depression carries the graver risk than treatment with Prozac.

Nevertheless, it is very likely that many seriously depressed adults, and parents of hyperactive children, have been understandably, and unnecessarily, frightened by negative, sensational reports in the media.

The fact is that there are several very discrete classes of psychiatric medications, and each class is quite different with regard to chemical composition, side effects, and potential for addiction. Not all psychiatric medications are tranquilizers. As an informed consumer it will be especially important for you to become knowledgeable about the various classes of medications, and to have accurate information regarding side effects, addiction potential, and so forth of the particular medication that is recommended for you or a member of your family.

Seeking Treatment

Who Can Prescribe Psychiatric Medications?

In most states the only people who can prescribe psychiatric medications are physicians and dentists (although for dentists, prescribing is limited to the dentist's scope of practice). In a few states such medications may be prescribed or furnished by appropriately trained nurse practitioners. Having the legal right to prescribe, however, does not imply that all such professionals are trained in the treatment of emotional and psychiatric disorders.

As noted in chapter 1, many prescriptions for psychiatric medications are written by primary care and family practice doctors. Some of these physicians are well trained in the diagnosis and treatment of emotional problems, and have years of experience carrying out such treatment. In fact, primary care physicians see between two and three people daily who are suffering from major depression. Lots of people visit their family doctor when they are experiencing psychological distress, for the three following reasons:

- First, they already have a relationship with their physicians and have learned to trust them.

- Second, many folks are reluctant to see a mental health professional (usually because of the negative stigma).

- Third, many psychiatric disorders cause significant physical symptoms (such as fatigue, aches and pains, sexual dysfunction, and insomnia) and thus may not even be recognized as emotional in origin, but are assumed by the patient to be symptoms of some sort of physical illness.

Although many people do seek psychiatric treatment from their primary care doctors, the ability to accurately diagnose psychiatric disorders in this setting is not good. This is the case primarily because of the fast-paced and brief nature of visits in a general medical clinic (the average office visit with a physician is between six and eight minutes!). While some physicians have developed ways to accurately identify their patients' psychological problems, some studies show that as many as 50 to 90 percent of the people who present with psychiatric disorders in a primary care setting either go undiagnosed or misdiagnosed (Jencks 1985; Gerber et al. 1989; Perez-Stable et al. 1990). Diagnosis and treatment of psychiatric problems in primary care settings are improving, but they still have a long way to go.

If you suspect that you (or a relative) are suffering from a psychiatric disorder and you want to consult your primary care doctor, it is strongly recommended that you first contact him or her and ask directly if they have experience in treating emotional disorders (e.g., depression or anxiety). Should your physician not have that experience, he or she is very likely to offer you a referral to a mental health specialist. If you are treated by your family practice doctor, we highly recommend that you also ask for the name of a psychotherapist. Psychiatric medication treatment is almost always more effective if taken in conjunction with psychotherapy.

Mental Health Specialists

Psychological treatment is available in most communities. Those who have special training in the diagnosis and treatment of psychological disorders include the following:

- Psychiatrists (M.D.)

- Psychologists (Ph.D., Psy.D., or Ed.D.)

- Clinical social workers (M.S.W. or L.C.S.W.)

- Licensed counselors (most have a master's degree: either an M.A. or M.S.)

- Some pastoral counselors

Although these professionals are all licensed to provide mental health treatment, their training and experience can vary tremendously. Thus, when seeking a referral for treatment, informed consumers should be sure to determine if a particular psychotherapist has the appropriate experience to provide the desired services.

In this book we provide a fairly comprehensive overview of psychiatric disorders. Clearly, our aim is not to make our readers into experts at diagnosis; even if that was our intention, we could not do that. We do feel, however, that it is important for you to know something about the particular problems you or a member of your family are experiencing. In part, this can help you to locate appropriate professional help.

Thus, after you have read the relevant chapter, if you believe, for example, that you are suffering from depression, it would be an excellent idea to make specific inquiries about a therapist's experience in treating depression. This can best be done by way of a telephone call. We strongly encourage people to speak to potential therapists by phone first, before making an appointment. This is a good way to find out important information about therapists (e.g., their availability, their areas of expertise, their fees, etc.). It will also give you a quick idea of how the therapist comes across. Many of our clients have remarked that the first telephone call made them feel more at ease and more confident that a particular therapist could help them. If you believe that psychiatric medication may be warranted in your treatment, it is entirely appropriate to ask therapists whether they use psychiatric medications as a part of their treatment approach. Also, it should be noted that some psychiatrists are trained primarily in psychopharmacology (medication treatment) and may not have any expertise in psychotherapy. Thus, it is also appropriate to ask potential psychiatrists if they provide psychotherapy in addition to medication treatment. If they do not, most of these doctors will be glad to provide the names of qualified therapists.

Of the mental health therapists listed above, only psychiatrists are licensed to prescribe medications. However, many nonmedical therapists (e.g., psychologists) work closely with psychiatrists or other physicians, and can provide psychological treatment in collaboration with that other doctor.

Finally, it is also important to note that pharmacists can be very helpful in providing you with information about prescriptions (especially about potential drug-drug interactions). Nowadays, many states mandate pharmacist consultation whenever a patient receives a new prescription or requires a change in an existing therapy. It is your right to receive this valuable information—take advantage of this resource!

Taking Positive Action: The Name of the Game

Almost all varieties of psychological disorders and emotional stress are accompanied by some feelings of powerlessness. Everyone in the throes of significant distress has tried their best to manage stress, and to a greater or lesser degree, has felt either frustrated or overwhelmed as the stress continues and the symptoms either persist or become worse. The main antidote for feeling powerless is to take action. For many thousands of people the first step in regaining control over their lives was taken when they decided to seek out mental health treatment. In a number of instances, that first step was a lifesaving decision. For many, many people it meant the difference between enduring months of suffering, as opposed to getting a treatment that effectively put them back on their feet.

If any one lesson has been learned, it is this: with major psychological disorders wishing, hoping, and gritting your teeth rarely work. And yet, only 25 percent of those with serious emotional problems look for help. Your decision to take your life seriously and take action to get treatment may not only be the smart thing to do, it is also a courageous act that is likely to be beneficial. It is also important to become an informed consumer. By knowing as much as you can about the diagnosis and treatment of psychiatric problems, you will be in the best position to find appropriate treatment. You have a right to ask any number of questions and to insist upon answers. This will be *your* treatment, *you* will be hiring the physician or therapist, and ultimately *you* will choose any and all of treatments that are recommended.

When you are informed about your choices, you will understand that you are calling the shots, and that you are in charge.

This understanding will help you to combat feelings of powerlessness. To use present-day lingo, knowledge is empowering.

Cosmetic Psychopharmacology

The term *cosmetic psychopharmacology* was coined by Dr. Peter Kramer, the psychiatrist and author of the best-selling book *Listening to Prozac* (1993). Dr. Kramer points out that most psychiatric medications were originally developed to treat the more severe mental and emotional disorders, such as schizophrenia, major depression, and bipolar disorder. And, in fact, a perusal of most psychiatric textbooks prior to the 1990s will reveal that this was clearly the major focus of psychiatric drug treatment. However, in the past decade, new discoveries were made that have broadened the focus of psychiatric medication treatment.

In particular, it has been found that some psychiatric medications are useful in treating the minor emotional disorders, such as mild depression, and even successful in changing what, heretofore, were thought to be aspects of personality (not disorders or diseases, per se). It is likely that these findings were made due to the following three factors.

1. First, many of the new drugs (especially the new generation of antidepressants) have very few side effects. Add to that the fact that antidepressants are nonaddictive and generally safe, even for long-term use, and it may come as no surprise that physicians have been willing to try these medications even on people who do not exhibit grave mental disorders.

2. A second factor has been the advent of managed care, with an increased emphasis on mandated brief treatment for psychiatric problems. It has been clear that many disorders (even minor adjustment disorders and stress reactions) require at least medium-length psychotherapy (i.e., a few months of therapy). Thus, some health insurers and others have advocated the use of psychiatric drugs (with or without psychotherapy) in an attempt to speed up treatment and recovery from a host of psychological woes. Although this is often a short-sighted maneuver, in fact, many people have responded well to this approach.

3. Finally, when patients were treated with psychiatric medications for more serious disorders, it was found that characteristics that

previously had been believed to be character traits (or aspects of temperament or personality) also appeared to change, sometimes significantly. For example, some patients treated for depression reported that in addition to experiencing relief from depression, they also noted changes in themselves—changes in their thinking, feeling, and behaving that they had never previously experienced. These changes included increased assertiveness, less social anxiety, a decreased tendency to fret and to worry, a more relaxed, casual approach to work, a less rigid approach to life, an enhanced ability for productivity, and so forth. Noticeable changes in the individual's personality also were observed. And, what may be the most interesting finding of all, many of these people reported that "this is my real self" (even though they may have never felt or acted that way in the past). This certainly raises all sorts of questions regarding how we define the "self." Is the self that set of personality characteristics that endures over the decades of life, or is it the more recent experiences (that simply "feel" better), such as boldness or feeling less inhibited in social settings?

Peter Kramer describes a number of cases in which people were treated not for major mental illnesses, but for what may be seen as personality quirks. And he invented the clever term "cosmetic psychopharmacology" to describe this particular use of psychiatric medications. Is it possible to use chemicals in the same way we might put on a "power tie" to wear to an important business meeting? Needless to say, this aspect of psychiatric medication treatment has sparked considerable controversy.

The use of these drugs for "cosmetic" purposes most likely accounts for some of the increase in the prescriptions for the newer generation of medications. In this book, however, we have chosen to focus on the most important targets for psychiatric medication treatment; namely, the serious and often debilitating psychological symptoms that accompany severe mental or emotional disorders. Suffice it to say that this is a complex matter of medical ethics and personal choice. For the moment, improving one's personality may be viewed as a possible positive side effect.

Emotions
and the Brain

In the Beginning

When modern psychiatry originated in the late 1800s, all psychiatrists were trained primarily in neurology (the study of diseases of the nervous system). The majority of psychiatrists of that time believed that serious mental illnesses (especially psychotic disorders such as schizophrenia and severe depression) were most likely caused by some kind of brain disorder or disease. In those days, because there were no effective treatments for serious mental illnesses, most patients were kept confined in asylums. Physicians of that time must have felt enormously frustrated and impotent, as they could do little to alleviate the intense suffering of those who were afflicted with psychiatric disorders. Thus, much time was spent in neuroanatomy laboratories studying the brains of deceased mental patients. The hunt was on for visible evidence of disease or trauma to the brain.

One important discovery was made then. It was found that many people suffering from very severe psychotic disorders were, in fact, experiencing the effects of syphilitic infection that had spread to the brain. (This was long before the development of antibiotics, so there were a large number of people so afflicted.) Beyond this one discovery, however, little else was learned about the brain or mental illness. Researchers were stumped, and millions of people worldwide continued to suffer, with no help in sight.

The Rebirth of Biological Psychiatry

During the first half of the twentieth century, psychiatry moved away from the biology lab and into the mental health clinic. Failure to find any promising leads in the realm of neurology led psychiatrists to explore a new, nonmedical approach for treating emotional problems: that approach was psychotherapy (or, as previously noted, what many called "talk therapy").

Psychotherapy was launched by the famous Austrian neurologist Sigmund Freud under the name of psychoanalysis. It, as well as a number of related disciplines, flourished during the first fifty or sixty years of the twentieth century. Although it had its limitations and certainly did not help everyone, it was rightly heralded as a breakthrough, because no other treatments existed. It was, in many ways, a godsend.

Psychotherapy had one limitation that immediately became apparent to most mental health professionals; the very severe mental illnesses did not respond well at all to psychotherapeutic techniques. In one of his last papers, Freud (1940) wrote that he believed eventually it would be discovered that the most severe disorders (e.g., schizophrenia) are caused by some kind of brain malfunction. He speculated further that one day researchers would find medications that would prove helpful in treating these very severe disorders.

That breakthrough arrived in the early 1950s. In 1954, purely by accident, it was found that a drug being used to reduce the adverse effects of general anesthesia also had antipsychotic properties. When this medication (now known by the trade name of Thorazine) was given to people suffering from chronic schizophrenia for several weeks, there were dramatic changes in their behavior. The drug tranquilized very agitated patients and, more importantly, it was often effective in reducing hallucinations and greatly improving the patients' ability to think logically and coherently.

When viewed in an historical context, this discovery was truly a miraculous finding. In the years before the discovery of Thorazine, most seriously disturbed patients were relegated to lifetime confinement in state mental hospitals. These hospitals, often referred to as "snake pits," were grim, bleak repositories for thousands of lost souls. By 1955, for the first time, the populations of mental hospitals began to decline, as many patients improved enough to be able to return to their families and communities.

Human beings who had been completely out of touch with consensual reality, who were badly regressed and beyond hope, were coming back to life. And, somehow, this remarkable change was due to specific chemical molecules producing some type of change in brain functioning. These early drugs also had side effects (sometimes serious) and, clearly, the medications did not "cure" schizophrenia. But it was undeniable that the drugs did make a significant difference and, for the first time, there was hope that treatments could be developed to help those who had suffered so much.

The fact that chemicals could so alter psychiatric symptoms ignited a growing interest in brain functioning and mental illness. Remember, the first psychiatric drug (and several others thereafter) was discovered only by accident. Early researchers had no true understanding about how these medications worked, but they quickly began to speculate. And the search was on, once again, to find out more about the biology of emotional and mental illness.

The Decade of the Brain

A multitude of theories were proposed and, as is the case in all areas of science, many of those theories were ultimately rejected. Nevertheless, investigations continued at a frantic pace. A good deal of the research was supported by pharmaceutical companies. By the mid-'70s, psychiatric drugs were among the top money-makers in the pharmaceutical industry. Besides the introduction of antipsychotics, drugs were also developed to treat anxiety, depression, and bipolar (manic-depressive) disorder. And, gradually, the newer medications proved more effective and less likely to have debilitating side effects than the earlier drugs. Research in the neurosciences was invigorated by the development of exciting new technologies. Innovations included the following new high-tech tools:

- CT (computerized tomography) and MRI (magnetic resonance imaging) scans (sophisticated devices for photographing the human brain)

- PET (positron emission tomography) and SPECT (single photon emission computerized tomography) scans (which allow

the researcher to watch actual metabolic functioning as it occurs in the living brain), and

• Gene mapping

President George Bush designated the 1990s as the "decade of the
brain," and rightly so; in that decade knowledge about brain functioning took a quantum leap.

The Basic Brain

The following discussion presents some very basic concepts
about the brain that will help you to understand more about the
biology of emotional and mental disorders. Of course, a comprehensive discussion of these topics is beyond the scope of this
book; however, at the end of the book there are some excellent
references for readers interested in a more extensive discussion.

It may be helpful to think of the brain as organized in layers
or levels. Neuroscientist Robert Ornstein (1984) uses the metaphor
of a ramshackle house to describe the organization. Imagine a
small and very basic house has just been built. Some years later, a
few rooms are added to the basic structure. And, a few years later,
even more additions are constructed. The original house is not
torn down; it is still there and still intact, but more and more modern rooms have been added to the basic structure. So it is with the
human brain.

The Reptilian Brain

In human beings, the oldest and most basic parts of the brain
are called the brain stem, hind-brain, and mid-brain. (These parts
are analogous to the first story of the ramshackle house.) The
structure and functioning of these parts of the brain are identical
to those found in many lower species. In particular, they are similar to the brain of reptiles. Thus, these parts of the brain are sometimes referred to as the "reptilian brain." The reptilian part of the
brain monitors a number of vital functions necessary for life, including heart rate, breathing, blood pressure, and so forth.

The Central Core of the Brain

The second story of this biological house is represented by
the central core of the brain. It contains two important brain centers: the hypothalamus and the limbic system.

Functions of the Hypothalamus

The first important part of the brain's central core is a tiny structure called the hypothalamus. This pea-sized but very complex structure controls or influences a number of important biological functions such as, control of biological drives like sex, hunger, and thirst; control of biological rhythms that influence sleep cycles and energy levels; influence on the immune system's functions; site of the "pleasure centers," and important in other emotional experiences.

A number of psychiatric disorders are thought to involve a malfunction of the hypothalamus. Such malfunctions can result in symptoms like insomnia, significant fatigue, appetite loss or increase, decreased sex drive, and in some instances, an impaired immune system, which can result in poor health and decreased resistance to disease.

Functions of the Limbic System

The second important group of brain structures found in the central core of the brain, surrounding the hypothalamus, are collectively referred to as the limbic system. The limbic system is commonly called the "emotional brain," and for good reason. These structures play a very important role in two aspects of emotional behavior. The first is that they are, in a sense, the launching pad for felt emotions. Thus, when you feel angry or afraid, this experience is set in motion by chemical activity taking place in one or more of the brain structures of the limbic system.

A second way the limbic system contributes to emotional behavior is that certain parts of the system operate as emotional control centers; that is, they play an important role in inhibiting and controlling emotional actions. For instance, at one time or other, we all have been treated rudely by another person. In such moments, it is perfectly understandable to become irritated or angry. However, for a number of good reasons, most of us do not punch out the offending person. We find a way to contain and hold our anger in check.

The ability to accomplish this type of self-control depends in part on the appropriate functioning of one of several structures in the limbic system. Most major psychiatric disorders involve some loss of emotional control (e.g., anger is being "out of control"; intense sadness is experienced as engulfing). Evidence is accumulating suggesting that this loss of control can often be traced to subtle, but important malfunctions in the limbic centers. It should come as no surprise to learn that the limbic system is the locale in the brain where most psychiatric medications appear to do their work.

The Cortex

The cortex is the highest level of the brain. It exists in many animals, but in most species it is relatively undeveloped, with the exception of primates (monkeys, apes, and humans). The cortex is the site of perception, information processing, thinking, reasoning, and all the higher human cognitive abilities. One part of the cortex deserves special attention: the frontal lobes.

The Frontal Lobes

In terms of human evolution, the frontal lobes are thought to be the most recent and advanced addition to the brain. (In the metaphor, the frontal lobes would be the penthouse, or the last room added to the basic house.)

A number of important functions are associated with the frontal lobes (in particular, the pre-frontal cortex, the front half of the frontal lobes). Those functions include: inhibiting emotional reactions, maintaining attention and concentration, and thinking complex thoughts and problem solving.

The interconnections between the frontal lobes and certain limbic system structures are rich and complex. These brain areas work together to inhibit and control strong emotional reactions. One very common problem seen in those who have suffered serious damage to their pre-frontal cortex is the tendency to express very intense emotional reactions—especially irritability and anger. Such people may know that it is not appropriate to express anger in many situations and they may feel embarrassed or guilty after a display of aggression. They often report, however, that they find it very hard, if not impossible, to keep from lashing out in anger. Similarly, some people who have sustained injuries to the pre-frontal cortex notice that even mildly upsetting events can provoke intense sadness and floods of tears.

Other individuals, despite average or above average intelligence, exhibit difficulties maintaining focused attention and concentration, and they fail academically or occupationally. In some of these cases, the pre-frontal cortex has been implicated (i.e., in those suffering from Attention Deficit Disorder).

Disorganized thinking is the hallmark of schizophrenia. Although it is likely that many brain areas are involved in this terrible disorder, a great deal of research points to the role of the pre-frontal cortex, which has been shown to be extremely inactive (hypo-metabolic) in a number of people who were diagnosed as schizophrenic.

In another part of the frontal cortex (the lateral surface) malfunctioning can produce states of pronounced loss of vitality and decreased motivation (as is the case in some forms of major depression).

There is convincing evidence in a number of psychiatric disorders that the frontal cortex is dysfunctional. In most cases, the problem is not brain damage in the usual sense of the term, because the data suggests little evidence of actual tissue damage. The research findings do indicate, however, that problems can be traced to chemical abnormalities in these various regions of the brain. This brings us to another level of investigation—malfunctions at the level of the cell.

Brain Cells and Abnormal Chemistry

Normal brain functioning is dependent on the appropriate action of nerve cells (often called neurons). Each and every brain structure is made up of thousands, if not millions, of neurons. They are responsible for turning particular brain centers on and off. Somewhat akin to the way a television set works with electricity, some nerve cells carry energy that turns the system on, while others operate like a brake to slow it down or turn it off. In addition, a multitude of neurons carry out the fine-tuning of the system, much like the various control knobs on the TV set, which adjust for brightness, color, volume, and so forth. With more than one-hundred billion nerve cells, and over one-hundred trillion interconnections, it is amazing how well this incredibly complex system functions (at least most of the time).

The nerve cells that have been implicated as malfunctioning in various psychiatric disorders represent only about one percent of all brain neurons. Thus, when it is determined that a person has an emotional disorder that can be traced to a biological cause, one can assume that the vast majority of brain cells are functioning normally, and that the presumed malfunctions involve only a tiny percentage of the total brain cells. Yet, a dysfunction in these very few brain neurons can wreak havoc, resulting in intense suffering, marked disability, and, at times, life-threatening psychiatric problems.

How Nerve Cells Work

Every nerve cell functions by producing and releasing a particular chemical substance called a neurotransmitter. Sometimes these chemical substances are called "messenger molecules" because they influence other nerve cells and aid in the communication processes between nerve cells. Each nerve cell receives numerous messages from other nerve cells and subsequently sends messages to its neighboring, adjacent nerve cells. These chemical messages can have an impact on the functioning of an individual nerve cell. They can turn the cell on (causing the cell to fire a "nerve impulse"), they can apply brakes (causing the cell to become inactive), and they can sometimes cause an adjacent cell to produce and release hormones, or to grow or to die.

Remarkably, these very complex processes continue through all the decades of one's life. And, most of the time, they work well. But it is no surprise that the system can also break down. Let's look at a specific example.

The drug reserpine was used for a number of years to treat hypertension (high blood pressure). It was fairly effective for treating hypertension, but a number of people who took it became seriously depressed. In most instances, these people were emotionally mature, solid individuals with no history of mental illness or emotional problems. Yet some of them became suicidally depressed. Eventually, it was discovered that this intense reaction was caused by the effect that reserpine had on a very limited number of nerve cells situated in the limbic system and hypothalamus. When the drug was discontinued, the patients recovered from their depression. Antidepressant medications were also used and were effective in treating these patients' depressive symptoms.

Note: The neurotransmitting chemical that is released by a particular nerve cell is also the name given to that nerve cell. Thus, a dopamine nerve cell is a cell that manufactures and releases dopamine.

A number of chemical and environmental factors can derail the functioning of neurotransmitters. The list of nerve cells that have been implicated in major psychiatric disorders is growing. Currently, it includes the following:

- Serotonin (abbreviated 5-HT)
- Dopamine (DA)
- Norepinephrine (NE)
- Gamma-amino butyric acid (GABA) and
- Glutamate

Some of the factors that have been found to interfere with appropriate nerve cell functioning include the following:

- Specific medications (used to treat many illnesses)
- Recreational drugs (e.g., alcohol, cocaine)
- Hormonal fluctuations (especially female sexual hormones)
- A number of diseases that cause changes in body chemistry which interfere with brain functioning
- Stress (especially intense and prolonged stress)
- Genetic factors (Disorders believed to be caused by genetic vulnerability tend to run in families, and blood relatives may be at increased risk for developing the disorder.)

Since so many different factors can cause psychological symptoms, it is very important to obtain a thorough medical evaluation to rule out possible physical conditions or other causes that might contribute to current psychological symptoms.

Andy's Case

Andy is a fifty-four-year-old mechanic who was accompanied by his wife to the mental health clinic. He was so tense and anxious that his wife did most of the talking. "Doctor, I don't know what's wrong with my husband. He's never been this way before, but during the last six months he has become a bundle of nerves." Her description was accurate. Andy was incredibly rigid as he sat trembling in his chair. He too was perplexed by his problem. He reported feeling "very nervous all the time" and was plagued by insomnia and fitful, restless sleep.

As they talked, the therapist noted that Andy was using a nasal spray. The third time that Andy used the spray the therapist inquired about its use. Andy had begun to use it six months ago, during the hay fever season, and his use had continued well past that time of the year. To keep his nasal passages open, he found it necessary to use the spray many times each day. The decongestant was immediately suspect as the cause of his anxiety. Chronic over-use of nasal decongestants are known to cause anxiety symptoms. With his primary care doctor's help, Andy was able to wean himself from the nasal spray successfully. Two weeks later, he was himself again. "I thought that I was going nuts. It's hard to believe that a little nasal spray can change a man so much!"

How Psychiatric Medications Work

As mentioned in chapter 1, psychiatric medications are not all alike. In some cases, particular drugs are believed, in one sense, to "cure" the problem with certain malfunctioning nerve cells (i.e., to return the neurons to a state of normal functioning). Other medications do not result in lasting changes in cellular functioning, but rather operate to improve cell functioning temporarily (e.g., the medications may work when they are taken and will provide symptom relief but, if discontinued, the symptoms may return). In most cases, the goal of psychiatric medication treatment is to re-store the brain to a state of normal cellular functioning, which will contribute a great deal to reducing emotional suffering.

At the same time, no pills have ever been invented to mend broken hearts or to fill empty lives. No medication can teach peo-ple how to love one another, nor can drugs insulate us from some of the inevitable challenges and tragedies of life. One fact is clear, however, when the brain is not functioning appropriately, the task of dealing with difficult life circumstances is amplified enormously.

Getting "High" on Life: The Brain's Pleasure Centers

Neuroscientists have identified several places in the brain that are known as *pleasure centers*. These brain areas are a part of an internal, biological reward system. They have evolved to gener-ate emotional states that are experienced by people (and other ani-mals) as pleasant. Biologic pleasure centers are activated by the release of particular neurochemicals (e.g., dopamine, endorphins) that get "turned on" by certain kinds of life experiences. Under normal circumstances, events such as watching a funny movie, enjoying a tasty meal, or making love can evoke a whole range of feelings from joy, to a heightened sense of aliveness, to blissful euphoria. Pleasure centers can also be activated artificially. A person might have a completely awful and unsatisfying life, and yet may temporarily feel on the top of the world by drinking champagne or taking cocaine. (Of course, we are certainly *not* recommending this pathway to euphoria. There are significant risks in using alcohol and drugs.)

Conversely, in major depression, there is a considerable body of evidence that suggests the pleasure centers have become chemically inactivated. This results in a symptom known as *anhedonia* (an inability to experience either pleasure or a feeling of vitality). Thus, even if a wonderfully satisfying event were to take place in the life of a person with serious depression, it would most likely not cause any positive emotions at all. Typically, the response of the depressed individual would be to feel nothing. This is only one of the symptoms that make the life of a seriously depressed person so intolerably painful. Anhedonia has been likened to watching a sunset, but seeing no color. Fortunately, antidepressant medications have a good track record in bringing the pleasure centers back on line, as well as combating a variety of other depressive symptoms (see chapter 5).

Can Psychotherapy Change Brain Functioning?

This question has been subject to a good deal of speculation. In 1992, a now-classic study, performed by Baxter and colleagues, addressed the question by looking at the neurobiology of people suffering from obsessive-compulsive disorder (OCD) (see chapter 7). It had been found that people with severe OCD exhibited a specific metabolic abnormality in a particular part of the brain. This was revealed with the use of positron emission tomography (PET scan). In the study, a group of OCD patients was randomly assigned to two treatment groups. One group received standard drug treatment for OCD (serotonergic antidepressants—a proven treatment for OCD). The other group received a specialized form of psychotherapy (behavior therapy first employing exposure, and then response prevention). All the participants had evidence of their abnormal PET scans prior to treatment. After a number of weeks of treatment, both groups showed a significant amount of improvement in their obsessional symptoms. They were then evaluated by a second PET scan. Remarkably, *both* groups (those who received drugs and those who received only psychotherapy) demonstrated that brain functioning had normalized and no longer showed evidence of aberrant metabolism.

In studies of both humans and animals, negative experiences, such as prolonged, intense stress, have been demonstrated to cause marked changes in brain functioning. So it should come as no surprise that positive experiences might also affect brain functioning (i.e., improve it). The data, at this time, is limited but there is reason to believe that psychotherapy can alter brain functioning. The key element that may account for this, is the experience of mastery. Clearly, this was one result of Baxter's study of OCD (1992).

When those patients began treatment, many of them had intense fears of dirt and germs, but after treatment they were able to work and function in dirty environments (i.e., to clean a toilet) and to face similar situations with much less fear. Many reported that they felt more in control of their lives and an enhanced sense of mastery. Extensive research on the effects of psychotherapy indicates that the common element in the various forms of psychotherapy is an increased sense of mastery and self-control (Bandura 1991). We eagerly await additional research that may shed more light on this theory.

Managing Your Medications

The material presented in this chapter is very general. By no means does it describe all of the complex interactions that take place within the human body when medications are taken. Our intention is not to provide detailed information as a textbook would, but rather to describe and explain some extremely important principles that you can use to make sure you get the most benefit out of your medications. By understanding the factors that can affect how a medicine acts in your body, you will be more capable of providing your doctor with accurate information to guide him or her in selecting the right drug for you at the right dose. Be sure to ask your doctor or pharmacist for specific information that you think might be important to help you understand your medicines better.

Medications: An Historical Perspective

In modern medicine, medications play a fundamental role in the treatment of most diseases or symptoms. This has not always been the case. Prior to the early 1900s there were relatively few useful medicines available. Breakthrough discoveries and technological advances in this century have provided the tools to better understand human physiology, and to produce purer and more reliable medications. It is important to recognize that even as sophisticated as our knowledge of drugs is at the present time, there is still a great deal we do not know about them. A quick glance through any standard pharmacology reference will confirm this statement. In discussions about medicines used to treat psychiatric conditions, it is especially important to keep in mind that there are limits to existing knowledge. Even though there have been tremendous strides in understanding how the brain works, we still do not have the capability to measure all of its functions.

Conversely, because of our modern sophisticated technology, it is tempting to assume that we know exactly what effects a drug will have on the body. Today, new biological discoveries are made and new drugs are developed at a remarkable pace. There may be a tendency to accept each new development as the final and best answer to long-standing questions regarding human behavior and mental health conditions. It is important, however, to maintain a healthy skepticism until new information has been confirmed over some period of time, or until new drugs have produced a well-established record of safety and effectiveness. Even the most rigorous clinical trials do not approximate all the effects of the wide use of a drug in diverse populations after it has been released into the marketplace (Nies 1990).

Psychopharmacology deals primarily with drugs intended to help symptoms that are categorized under the three main types of disorder: (1) mood, such as depression; (2) anxiety; and (3) psychotic disorders, such as schizophrenia. The use of these medications is relatively recent, with widespread use not beginning until the '50s and '60s. Since then the commercial growth of psychiatric drugs has been phenomenal, which indicates how commonly these conditions occur and how great the need is to treat them. Much of the basic research aimed at understanding how psychiatric medications work has added to the overall knowledge-base of emotional and mental illnesses.

How Medications Work: Basic Pharmacology

At a very basic level, pharmacology is the science of dealing with the process of how drugs interact with the body to produce certain effects. Included in the study of pharmacology is knowledge about the origins and chemical properties of drugs, as well as a thorough understanding of the biology and chemistry of the body. A *drug* is broadly defined as "any chemical that affects living processes" (Benet, Mitchell, and Sherner 1990). The actions that drugs take extend from the microscopic or molecular level, to individual organs such as the heart and brain, to the body as a whole organism.

Drugs and Receptors

At the molecular level, most drugs interact with specific receptors to produce their therapeutic effects. Receptors are structures located on the outside surface of nerve cells that interact with a variety of chemicals, including medications. To understand the interaction, an often-used analogy is drawn between that of a lock and key, where the receptor acts as the lock and the chemical as the key. There are various drug receptor systems located throughout the body.

Side Effects

The effects of drugs can be those that are intended, called the *therapeutic* effects, or unintended, thought of as *side effects*. Although side effects often are bothersome and sometimes create serious problems, some side effects actually can be beneficial. Many side effects are most noticeable when a medication is first started, or when the dose is increased. Most diminish over time. However, side effects that persist or get worse should never be ignored.

The published information about a given drug's side effects is fairly extensive. Generally, when reading about a medication's side effects you will note that they are categorized by how often they occur. Usually these groupings of side effects are designated as: frequent or common, infrequent, or rare.

In Part II of this book, *The Consumer's Guide to Psychiatric Drugs,* we cover most of the common side effects and most of the infrequent and rare side effects that could be potentially serious. Since we do not reproduce all of the literature that drug manufacturers are required to report, our lists are not all-inclusive. We do provide the most important information you need in order to benefit from the medication your doctor has prescribed. If you have any questions about the side effects of the medication you are taking, you should consult your doctor.

Basic Pharmacokinetics

To better understand and benefit from medications of any type it is important to have a working knowledge of some of the processes that take place when medications are ingested. The principles summarized in the following pages apply to medications in general. It is important to remember, however, that every person is biologically unique. And even though medications generally follow somewhat predictable patterns, it is obvious that some people will react differently to the same medication than others.

Once a drug enters the body, a cascade of actions is set in motion. Certain bodily organs or systems can produce various effects on a medication. There are four basic processes that occur: *absorption, distribution, metabolism,* and *excretion.* Collectively these processes are called *pharmacokinetics.* What follows is a very brief description of these four functions, intended to help you understand the complexities involved in predicting how medicines act in the body.

Absorption

Most drugs are absorbed in the stomach or small intestine. The presence of food, milk, or other medications in the stomach can affect a given medicine. It is important to find out how your medication should be taken with regard to meals. If the absorption of a medicine is known to be impaired when food is present in the stomach, then it might be advisable to take that medicine on an empty stomach. On the other hand, the presence of food sometimes increases the amount of a drug that is absorbed, in which case it might be preferable to take the medicine at mealtimes. Certain medications can irritate the stomach and should be taken with food or milk to lessen this effect and prevent damage to the stomach lining.

As a drug travels throughout the body it encounters various membranes that it must cross. One of the most important of these barriers is called the *blood-brain barrier.* This barrier serves to limit the substances that pass into the brain. It is one of the ways the body protects the brain from damage caused by chemicals or other toxins. Some medications pass freely into the brain, while others have more limited accessibility.

The total amount of a medication that is ingested may not equal the amount that ultimately becomes available at the place in body for which it is intended. This is a principle called *bioavailability*. For example, if a medication is known to break down and be inactivated by the acidic environment of the stomach, only a certain percentage of the original dose will reach the bloodstream. In this case, less than 100 percent of the drug will be bioavailable. In contrast, a drug injected directly into the bloodstream is considered to be nearly 100 percent bioavailable because it reaches the bloodstream intact.

Bioavailability is also the benchmark measure used to compare products made by different manufacturers, or between generic and brand-name products. With most generic drugs, bioavailability closely matches that of the original brand-name product. Such generic products can provide an economical advantage over higher-cost brand-name drugs. Certain medications, however, are not readily formulated into generic products and the brand-name product may be superior. From a practical standpoint, it may be more important not to make frequent switches between products.

Distribution

Once a medication reaches the bloodstream it is then distributed to various areas or organs in the body. The distribution pattern varies from drug to drug. For most medicines, the distribution process is very straightforward; for others, the pattern is more complex. For example, more complicated processes apply to medicines that are preferentially stored in fatty areas of the body. A drug can remain for long periods of time in fatty areas, somewhat like being stored in a reservoir. When in these storage areas, the drug is not readily available to produce any action; rather, it has been deposited and is inactive.

The amount of medicine in the reservoir will vary in order to reach a balance with the amount that is in the bloodstream. If the amount in the bloodstream drops, then some of the medicine will be released from the storage area. If the amount in the bloodstream is stable and adequate, none will be released from the storage area, and the amount in the reservoir can continue to accumulate.

For people taking antidepressants and antipsychotics, understanding how drug distribution works can be very important. To a large degree, these types of medicines are stored in fatty areas.

This means that even after a medication is discontinued, because some of it has been stored, it will gradually re-enter the bloodstream until all of it is eliminated from the body. In such instances, there can be continuing effects from the medication for several weeks or longer after it has been discontinued.

This is very important information to remember about stopping antidepressants or antipsychotics. In essence, a person can continue to experience the benefits, or side effects, of the medicine even though it is not being taken as a daily dose. After stopping, the symptoms may return several weeks down the road. It is important to watch out for signs that symptoms might be returning, not just in the first few days after stopping a medicine, but for as long as eight weeks after discontinuing.

Metabolism

This process, which occurs primarily in the liver, is also known as *biotransformation*. Most medications are metabolized, or chemically altered, to varying degrees by the liver. The actual process takes place through the action of enzymes that break down molecules from their original size to smaller ones that then can be eliminated by the kidney more easily.

The extent and rate of metabolism for a given drug is generally consistent, within a range, from person to person. However, some people may be exceptionally fast metabolizers while others may be especially slow. In these instances, there is less predictability when determining the dose or frequency of a given drug, and adjustments are often necessary. Slow metabolizers, for instance, might be extremely sensitive to the side effects of a medication, even at a low or average dose. Antidepressants and antipsychotics are classes of medications that are especially prone to differences in metabolizing capability. There is some evidence that there may be a genetic influence in those who are slow metabolizers.

People who have damaged livers may have impaired metabolic ability, which can lead to a buildup of medication in the body. To prevent serious side effects from excessively high levels of a medication in the blood, it may be necessary for such people to take smaller amounts of medicine, or less frequent doses.

Because the liver is called upon to metabolize most medications, there are times when multiple drugs will compete for the same enzymes. This competition is the source of one of the most common types of drug interactions. Usually one drug wins this contest over the other. The result is that one medication will build up in the body because the liver is busy metabolizing the other. Adjusting the dose of one or both of the interacting medications may become necessary.

Excretion

Excretion is the second step in the process by which drugs are eliminated from the body. The first step, metabolism, happens via the liver as described above. Excretion takes place primarily through the kidneys. If there is kidney damage, medications can accumulate to higher than desired (or even dangerous) levels. If the kidneys are working in a less than ideal manner, adjustments in medication may be necessary to avoid unnecessary or dangerous side effects.

Half-Life

A measure of a medication's action that is related to excretion is called half-life. The *half-life* is the amount of time required for the blood level of a drug to drop by 50 percent. A drug's half-life is used to decide how often it should be taken and also to determine correct dosages. For instance, drugs with short half-lives will require more doses throughout a twenty-four-hour period because they will leave the body faster. Medicines with longer half-lives will not need to be taken as frequently because they will stay in the body longer.

Getting the Most out of Your Medications

Getting the maximum benefit from your medicines requires that you and your doctor work together. Your doctor will ask many specific questions before prescribing a medication. The following list highlights some of the key steps you can take to work effectively with your doctor in managing your medicines.

What Your Doctor Needs to Know

Your doctor will need the following information: Your complete medical history; everything to which you are allergic; the names and dosages of all the medicines you take, including over-the-counter products; your past experiences with medicines, positive and negative; how much alcohol you drink on a daily or weekly basis; all the recreational drugs that you use.

What You Can Do to Manage Your Medicines

Take the medicine exactly as prescribed. Taking more than prescribed can be dangerous. Missing doses can mean you don't get better. If you do not understand the directions, ask your doctor or pharmacist to clarify them for you. If you have trouble remembering to take your medicine, ask someone like a family member or health care provider to help you set up a system.

Be sure you understand exactly why you are taking a given medication. If your questions are not answered to your satisfaction, be persistent with your doctor or pharmacist to get the information you need. This is your right.

Understand how long it should take to begin to feel better. Do not hesitate to contact your doctor if you experience unexpected side effects or if you are not getting better in a reasonable time.

Avoid seeing too many different doctors who might prescribe many kinds of medicine. If you have an established need to see several physicians, be sure each doctor is aware of what the other doctors are prescribing for you.

If you are having difficulties taking a medicine because it is hard to swallow, find out whether it is available in a liquid form. Also, some tablets are suitable for crushing, and the contents of some capsules can be mixed in a liquid. Check with your doctor or pharmacist first.

Read the label on the medicine bottle every time you take a dose to be sure you are taking the correct medication. Some people have many bottles of medicine and they can be mixed up easily. Become familiar with what your medicine looks like. If you receive a prescription that doesn't "look right" to you, be sure to double-check it with your pharmacist. Never take your medicine in the dark when you cannot see exactly what you are swallowing.

Do not switch medication bottles. Keep your medicine in the original bottle in which it came. Never put all your medicines together in one bottle. If you need help in keeping your medicines straight, there are pill reminder boxes that you can purchase to help you keep track.

Make sure you put the lids back on tightly. By law, child-resistant lids are required for prescription medicines to prevent children from accidental poisonings. Some adults find these hard to use and will compensate by not putting the lids on securely. Such people can ask for a waiver and receive lids that are not child-resistant. In any case, it is essential to prevent ingestion by children because accidental overdoses can be fatal to them.

Know whether your prescription has refills. Sometimes your doctor will want to check with you before authorizing your refills. Keep track of when you are close to running out of your medicine and allow ample time to get your refills. Be familiar with how to get your prescriptions refilled. Sometimes people run into problems getting refills and will go for several days without taking their medicine. In that amount of time it is possible for symptoms to return. Taking medicine consistently, without any lapses in treatment, is the best way to ensure that you (or your loved one) will get better—and stay that way.

Follow the storage instructions. In general, most drugs should be kept in a cool, dry place, away from high temperatures, in an area of low humidity and out of direct light. In actuality, the bathroom "medicine" cabinet is one of the worst places to store your medications because of the humidity and temperature of the bathroom. If you have not stored you medicine appropriately, it may deteriorate or undergo a physical change to become a harmful chemical.

Do not take medications past the expiration date on the bottle. The expiration date is accurate, assuming that proper storage instructions were followed.

Keep taking your medicines as prescribed. Sometimes people decrease their dosage or discontinue their medication altogether because the cost is prohibitive. However, taking less that an adequate dose, won't provide the relief that is sought. If you are unable to afford an expensive medicine, your doctor and pharmacist will often work with you to find a more affordable drug. If you do not have insurance that pays for your prescriptions, try to get an idea of how much your medicines will cost you each month.

Useful Tips About Psychiatric Medications

If the treatment of your mental health condition requires medication, there is a lot you can do to make sure you get better. Do not view the prescribing of your medicine as a passive process. Your doctor's decision is based not only on his or her observations and examination of you, but also on your ability to provide complete and honest information. No matter how insignificant a concern or question might seem to you, it is important that your doctor hear what is on your mind.

Be open with your doctor if you have not been taking your medicine as prescribed. The doctor will try to work with you to figure out why you are having problems with it. Sometimes, when people are depressed, they may have trouble remembering whether they took their medication. Some people may feel so bad about themselves that they don't believe they deserve to get better. Others might feel so hopeless about their chances of recovery that they have little faith in the medicine working. All of these possibilities are typical in a depression. Your doctor will understand the difficulties you face and help you work through them.

Some people will be fearful of taking medicines to treat depression, anxiety, or psychotic disorders. If you are afraid in this regard, share your concerns with your doctor. In some cases these concerns are based on faulty information or misconceptions. Your doctor or pharmacist can provide you with factual information that can clear up any misunderstandings and often will allay your fears.

Occasionally, some people become suspicious of everyone and everything involved in their treatment, especially if their problem is a psychotic disorder such as schizophrenia. At those times, people may think that their medicine is intended to harm them or that someone can change their medicine in such a way as to "poison" them. In these situations it can be quite difficult to provide reassurance.

If you have ever thought this way, or if you have a loved one who thinks this way, it is important to know that prescription medications are manufactured under very tight quality control conditions. It would be nearly impossible for an individual doctor, nurse, or pharmacist to change the ingredients in a prepared tablet or capsule. In addition, most medications are required by law to have clear identifying markings on them. If you are familiar with what your medicine normally looks like, you'll be able to notice immediately if you receive something else.

Medications have an established role in the treatment of most mental health conditions. They can produce remarkable results and provide relief from the most painful and debilitating of symptoms. These drugs are among the most widely prescribed in the world and millions of people take them safely every day. There are abundant reasons to expect that your experience with these medications will be positive and that you will find relief from your symptoms.

Depression

Introduction

Many people occasionally will say that they feel *depressed*. This can refer to a host of unpleasant emotions such as feeling "blue," moodiness, feelings of sadness, disappointment, discouragement, being unmotivated, or just feeling "out of sorts." For most of us, feeling down in the dumps occasionally or being saddened temporarily is a normal part of human life. These are understandable reactions to a myriad of difficult life experiences.

In the United States, however, every year 10 percent of the population experiences a much more devastating mood disorder, referred to these days as either *major depression* or *clinical depression*. Over the life span of the average American the prevalence of major depression is even higher, affecting 19 percent—one out of five Americans will at some point in their lives suffer with this form of severe emotional disorder (Kessler et al. 1994). With such a high incidence, it is hard to imagine that anyone has not either experienced depression personally or known close friends or relatives who have had episodes of clinical depression. The bottom line—major depression is an extremely common experience.

Major depression differs from minor bouts of sadness in a number of ways that are discussed in detail later in this chapter. However, its main characteristics are as follow:

- It is extremely severe.
- If not treated, it generally lasts for months.

- It often results in significant disability. (In addition to tremendous personal suffering, during episodes of major depression, otherwise capable people often cannot function at work or in school, marriages fall apart, and loving parents find it nearly impossible to nurture and guide their children.)
- Rates of alcohol and other types of substance abuse are higher.
- For untreated or undertreated people, there is a risk of suicide (the lifetime mortality risk from suicide is 15 percent) (Hamilton 1989, 897).
- Chronic depression contributes to poor physical health.

Clinical depression is obviously much more than a mere case of the blues. It is a common and often devastating emotional illness. The real tragedy is that only one-third of those experiencing a major depression ever receive treatment. Most of these people somehow grit their teeth and suffer for months and months (the average length of an episode of depression is from nine to fifteen months, unless treated). Yet, according to the National Institute of Mental Health, 80 percent or more of those experiencing major depression can be successfully treated, and in many cases symptom relief can occur in a matter of weeks (NIMH, D/ART Fact Sheet 1990).

This high rate of treatment success is due to the development of several effective types of therapy, including some types of psychotherapy (e.g., cognitive therapy or interpersonal therapy) and medical treatments, which are discussed in detail later in this chapter.

A Recurring Illness

For a third of people experiencing a major depression, the current episode will be a once in a lifetime event. However, for about two-thirds of these people, unfortunately, the disorder will recur (APA 1994a, 341). In this group, many will experience ongoing, chronic depression, while most will be plagued with recurring episodes of the illness. Although this may sound bleak, the good news is that medical treatments for depression also have been shown to be very effective in preventing relapse. Thus, when considering treatment for depression, it is important to focus not only on resolving the current episode but also on taking steps to prevent recurrence of the disorder. We will focus on relapse prevention in this chapter, as well.

Not Everyone Will Understand

It is a very common experience for those going through a depression to hear comments from concerned friends or family that reveal the concerned person does not truly understand the nature of clinical depression. For example, people make statements like these: "You just need to look on the bright side." "Just try to snap yourself out of it." "You need to try harder—you need to pull yourself up by your bootstraps." They may even say, "Don't worry—be happy." Their intentions may be good, but they simply do not understand.

True clinical depression drags people into a kind of emotional paralysis from which it is difficult to escape, despite considerable effort. It must be emphasized that depression can affect anyone from any walk of life. It knows no social or economic barriers. It can occur to anyone regardless of the level of intelligence or strength of character. During the past two decades, a number of discoveries were made in the medical and neurological sciences that have helped us to understand more about the role the brain plays in emotional disorders. This is especially true when it comes to understanding the underlying, biological basis of some types of depression. And, as a result of these discoveries, the medical treatments for depression have improved enormously. Nevertheless, it is important to consider several concerns that have been raised regarding psychiatric medications.

Making the Diagnosis

Before looking at diagnosis per se, it is important to understand the distinctions between three human experiences: reactive sadness, grief, and clinical depression. *Reactive sadness* is an experience common to most human beings. It is considered a normal, healthy emotional reaction to minor losses and disappointments. This kind of sadness is very transient, lasting only several minutes, a few hours, or, at most, a few days. It is unpleasant, but typically does not interfere with one's functioning. People feel sad, but they can continue to work, to raise their kids, and to go about the tasks of everyday life. Normal, minor bouts of sadness do not knock people off of their feet.

In contrast, *grief* is a much more intense and sometimes devastating human experience. However, it is considered a normal and, most likely, inevitable emotional reaction that people in every culture across the world experience in the aftermath of a major loss (e.g., the death of a loved one, or a divorce). Grief tends to have a major disruptive effect on the lives of sufferers and can result in prolonged periods of sadness, mourning, and loneliness. Mental health professionals make a distinction between what is called uncomplicated bereavement and complicated grief reactions. *Uncomplicated bereavement* is considered a very painful, albeit healthy, normal response to a major loss. It often results in a prolonged period of mourning, which can last anywhere from a few months to several years. We want to emphasize that normal grieving may last a very long time; broken hearts do not mend quickly. On the other hand, *complicated grief reactions* become especially severe and can disintegrate into clinical depression.

The essential feature is of uncomplicated bereavement is that it seems to be a necessary part of emotional healing, (i.e., that some amount of mourning seems to be necessary for people to come to terms with major losses). There are two other important features that separate uncomplicated bereavement from the kind of grief that turns into clinical depression. The first is that, during normal grieving, despite tremendous personal suffering, the grieving person's self-esteem and sense of self-worth remain relatively intact. This is not the case with the complicated grief that becomes major depression. Almost always, in more severe depressions, grieving people experience a significant erosion in their sense of self-worth.

The second marker is a set of symptoms commonly a part of major depression that is *absent* in uncomplicated bereavement. When the following symptoms are seen in the midst of grief, it is likely that the grieving process has become derailed; in addition to mourning, the person has slipped into major depression: Grief becomes depression when there is significant agitation*, early morning awakening*, serious weight loss*, suicidal ideation or attempts, anhedonia (loss of the ability to experience any pleasure)*, and marked impairment of social, interpersonal, academic, or occupational functioning.

---

* When this clinical picture emerges, psychotherapy, psychotropic medication treatment, or both, become necessary. The symptoms marked with an asterisk are targets for antidepressant medications.

The vast majority of individuals encountering major losses grieve, but do not become seriously depressed and do not need psychological or psychiatric treatment. However, it has been found that about 25 percent of those experiencing a major loss will, in fact, go on to develop clinical depression (complicated grief reactions), and certainly may need and benefit from mental health treatment (Zisook 1996). In these cases, the depression must be resolved before people can begin to come to terms with their painful loss adequately. Medication treatment may be indicated when grief turns into depression.

Clinical depressions are characterized by their intensity, duration, impact on functioning, and a host of specific symptoms that are outlined below.

How Depression Is Diagnosed

There has been a great deal of media attention during recent years regarding the biological basis of depression (often referred to as a type of chemical imbalance in the brain). Thus, one might assume that there now are laboratory tests to diagnose depression. However, at the time this is being written, such tests are used only for research purposes and not clinical settings. Currently, the diagnosis of depression is based on three main sources of data: the particular signs and symptoms, the patient's own history (e.g., the onset of symptoms and any history of prior depressions), and the patient's family history of emotional problems.

Signs and Symptoms of Depression

It is useful to consider two main sets of depressive symptoms. The first set is referred to as Core Symptoms, which are symptoms that are seen in nearly all types of depression.

Core Symptoms Common to All Depressions

- Mood of sadness, despair, emptiness
- Anhedonia (loss of the ability to experience pleasure)
- Low self-esteem

- Apathy, low motivation, and social withdrawal
- Excessive emotional sensitivity
- Negative, pessimistic thinking
- Irritability
- Suicidal ideas

Note: Some degree of decreased capacity for pleasure (anhedonia) may be seen in all types of depression. In depressions that involve a biochemical disturbance, this loss of ability to experience pleasure can become so pronounced that the patient experiences almost no moments of joy or pleasure. Such people are said to have a "nonreactive mood," which means that they are unable to get out of their depressed mood even temporarily.

A second group of symptoms are called the *biological* or *physical symptoms* of depression (in psychiatric literature these are also referred to as *vegetative* symptoms). As will be discussed shortly, some types of depression are believed to involve significant changes in physical functioning. The biological symptoms of depression are listed below.

Biological Symptoms of Depression

- Appetite disturbance—decreased or increased, with accompanying weight loss or gain
- Fatigue
- Decreased sex drive
- Restlessness, agitation, or psychomotor retardation
- Impaired concentration and forgetfulness
- Pronounced anhedonia—total loss of the ability to experience pleasure
- Sleep disturbance—early morning awakening, frequent awakenings throughout the night; occasionally hypersomnia (excessive sleeping). Note that initial insomnia (difficulty in falling asleep) may be seen with depression, but is not diagnostic of a major depressive disorder. Initial insomnia can be seen with anyone experiencing stress in general. Initial insomnia alone is more characteristic of anxiety disorders than of depression

When a person is being evaluated for possible depression, the mental health professional (or primary care physician) should ask specifically about the presence or absence of these symptoms (both core symptoms and biological symptoms). Not all depressed people will have all of these symptoms, but they usually will have several at least. In general, for a diagnosis of depression to be made, such symptoms must be present for a period lasting at least two weeks.

Some types of depression appear to be associated with an underlying biological cause (a neurochemical disorder). In most cases these disorders tend to recur, and thus a history of prior episodes suggests that the disorder *may* be due, at least in part, to some form of biological vulnerability. Also, the more biologically based depressions tend to run in families. Consequently, obtaining a family history (to see if there are blood relatives who have had mood disorders or alcoholism) may provide important clues to the diagnosis. Depressions that include not only the core symptoms but also one or more of the biological symptoms, are likely to be caused by, at least in part, an underlying neurochemical disturbance. If there is also a history of prior episodes and/or a family history of depression, then the evidence is even stronger that biology may be involved. The reason this is important to determine is that those individuals for whom an underlying biological disorder is likely, also tend to be those who respond best to antidepressant medications.

Other Diagnostic Issues

Depression can be caused by many factors. Most of the time, they are a response to stressful life experiences, especially when people experience two major types of stressors. The first are losses: the loss of a loved one to death or divorce, the loss of a job, the loss of status, money, health, etc. The second group are life events that result in feelings of helplessness or powerlessness. When people encounter unrelieved and mounting stress they sometimes begin to think, "No matter what I do, I can't seem to solve these problems. . . ." Such a perception of powerlessness often provokes depression. In addition to life stresses certain biological changes can trigger depression. These include a number of physical diseases. These medical conditions often change body chemistry and ultimately affect the delicate chemical balance of the emotional brain.

Medical Disorders that Can Cause Depression

- Addison's disease
- Anemia
- Chronic fatigue syndrome
- Chronic pain
- Diabetes
- Hypothyroidism
- Influenza
- Malnutrition
- Porphyria
- Syphilis
- Ulcerative colitis

- AIDS
- Asthma
- Chronic infection (mononucleosis, tuberculosis)
- Congestive heart failure
- Cushing's disease
- Infectious hepatitis
- Malignancies (cancer)
- Multiple sclerosis
- Rheumatoid arthritis
- Systemic lupus erythematosus
- Uremia

When it is determined that a particular physical illness may, in fact, be causing depression, then the approach of choice generally is to focus on treating the particular disease (e.g., thyroid disease). When the disorder is successfully treated, typically depressive symptoms subside. At times, antidepressant medication and psychotherapy may also play an important role as part of the total treatment package. Additionally, a number of medications and recreational drugs commonly *cause* depression.

Drugs that Can Cause Depression

Type	Generic name	Brand-Name
• Alcohol	Wine, beer, spirits	Various brands
• Antianxiety drugs	Diazepam	Valium
	Chlordiazepoxide	Librium
• Antihypertensives	Reserpine	Serpasil, Ser-Ap-Es
(for high blood	Propranolol	Inderal
pressure)	hydrochloride	
	Methyldopa	Aldomet
	Guanethidine sulfate	Ismelin sulfate
	Clonidine hydrochloride	Catapres
	Hydralazine hydrochloride	Apresoline hydrochloride

- Antiparkinsonian   Levodopa   Sinemet
  drugs   carbidopa
                      Levodopa   Dupar, Larodopa
                      Amantadine   Symmetrel
                        hydrochloride

- Birth control pills   Progestin-estrogen   Various brands
                        combination

- Corticosteroids   Cortisone acetate   Cortone
  and other   Estrogen   Premarin, Ogen,
  hormones   Estrace,
                                                 Estraderm
                      Progesterone   Provera, Depo-
                        and derivatives   Provera,
                                                 Norlutate,
                                                 Norplant,
                                                 Progestasert

The majority of people treated with these medications do not experience depression, although a small percentage do. If there have been no major stressful life events in recent times, and the depressive symptoms emerged in the weeks following the beginning of treatment with these medications, then the drug may be suspect as a cause of depression. If you or a family member are receiving medical treatment, and are taking one of the drugs listed and have become depressed, it is important not to discontinue the medication; rather you should contact your physician and share your concerns with him or her.

Alcohol

Alcohol is one of the most common drugs to cause depression and deserving of special attention. It has been definitively shown that for many individuals alcohol can, by itself, cause serious depressive reactions. Alcohol is, however, a seductive drug: many people certainly notice that minutes after drinking alcohol they feel more relaxed or experience a lifting of sadness or despair. Thus, the immediate effect is one of emotional relief. For this reason it is no surprise that when life becomes very stressful, a great many people turn to alcohol for some respite. This rapid and temporary relief is misleading, however, because over a period of weeks, ongoing alcohol use almost always worsens a depression.

Not only does alcohol directly cause depression, but daily, moderate-to-heavy alcohol use also interferes with the actions of antidepressant medications. Many individuals, who either failed to respond or experienced only partial relief when treated with antidepressants, were found to be using alcohol. In fact, this is one of the most common reasons that medical treatment for depression fails. Thus, it is *essential* that anyone suffering from depression who is also drinking alcohol discuss this with the therapist or physician. If treatment for depression is to be successful, alcohol use must be controlled.

Caution: If someone has been drinking a moderate-to-heavy amount of alcohol on a daily basis, abrupt discontinuation of medication can be dangerous. If you or a family member have been drinking a lot of alcohol, it is very important that your discontinuation be monitored medically.

Is a Medical Exam Necessary?

Because some depressions are triggered by underlying medical illnesses, it makes good sense to see your family physician to rule out possible medical causes. The exception to this is if the depression clearly emerged in the aftermath of a major, painful life event (e.g., a divorce, job loss, etc.). In any event, it may be wise to be seen by your physician, and nowadays, in the managed care system, most people need a mental health referral from their physician in any case.

Depression and the Brain

In the past two decades there were numerous advances in medicine and the neurosciences—new technologies and new discoveries. Now, it is widely accepted that in many if not most cases of clinical depression there are a number of well documented changes in brain functioning. Here are a few highlights of some important findings.

- Brain imaging techniques (PET and SPECT scanning) have revealed that in the majority of people suffering from major depression, the brain becomes significantly hypo-metabolic. (This means that the neurochemical activity of the brain falls well below normal levels of activity.) This does not occur throughout the brain, rather it affects primarily those parts that govern the ability to be self-motivated (e.g., the frontal cortex). The reduced activity in these regions is the likely cause of the apathy, low motivation, and loss of vitality that are common in most cases of clinical depression.

- Other findings reveal that in depression the hypothalamus (the part of the brain that regulates many biological drives and rhythms) is significantly dysfunctional. This accounts for a number of the biologically based symptoms discussed earlier, such as sleep disorders, loss of sex drive, pronounced fatigue, and changes in appetite. These brain abnormalities have been observed not only through brain imaging studies, but also in laboratory analyses of spinal fluid and measures of stress hormones.

- Current theory holds that such changes in brain functioning are due to abnormalities in two or three specific groups of nerve cells in the central nervous system. The brain is composed of 100 billion nerve cells and scores of different types of nerve cells make up the brain's incredibly complex organization. Interestingly, it is believed that only a tiny fraction of brain nerve cells are responsible for the biological malfunctions that underlie depression (probably only about one percent of the total nerve cells in the brain malfunction in depression).

- The three nerve cells believed to be implicated in major depression are: *serotonin (the scientific abbreviation for serotonin is 5-HT), norepinephrine (NE),* and *dopamine (DA).* (Nerve cells are named after the particular neurotransmitters they release; thus, nerve cells producing and secreting dopamine are called dopamine neurons.)

- All existing effective antidepressants are known to affect one or more of these classes of nerve cells, and, in general, restore their normal cellular functioning.

Types of Treatment

Treatments for depression can be divided into two classes: medical and nonmedical. We will briefly describe nonmedical approaches and then focus on medical treatments in detail.

For many years, people were treated for depression with psychotherapy (also called counseling or "talk therapy"). More recently, two specialized forms of psychotherapy were developed that now have fairly extensive studies documenting their effectiveness in treating depression. These are *cognitive therapy* and *interpersonal therapy.*

Psychotherapy is the treatment of choice for a mild-to-moderately severe depression, especially when the onset of the depression appears to be related to major life stresses. It is also a very important part of treatment for more severe depressions, although in more severe cases antidepressant medications may be the first-line treatment. Even when it is clear that the depression is directly due to a biochemical disorder or disease, psychotherapy is often essential to help the person learn how to cope with the disorder. It can also play an important role in successful relapse prevention.

Psychiatrists, psychologists, clinical social workers, and other licensed counselors provide psychotherapy. Such providers can be found by asking your family physician for a referral, contacting your local Mental Health Association, or looking in the Yellow Pages. Although most licensed psychotherapists do treat depression, it is a good idea when calling for an appointment to ask specifically whether the therapist has experience or special training in treating depression.

Treatments for depression fall into three classes: antidepressant medication treatments, light therapy, and electro-convulsive therapy (ECT).

The latter two approaches are discussed briefly toward the end of this chapter. Now, let's examine antidepressant medication treatment.

Antidepressants: What They Are and How They Work

It is very important to note that antidepressants are a specific and unique class of psychiatric medications; they are *not* tranquilizers and they are *not* stimulants. Antidepressants are believed to have their main effects on the aforementioned nerve cells—serotonin, norepinephrine, and/or dopamine. *As a rule, after several weeks of continued treatment, antidepressant medications restore these nerve cells to a state of normal functioning.* This point is worth emphasizing.

Some other drugs (like alcohol or tranquilizers) also can produce rather quick changes in one's feelings. However, such changes are truly "drug-induced effects"; and typically people feel "drugged" or at least know that "This feeling is not me—it's the drug." This is not the case with antidepressants. The changes experienced by those who respond to antidepressants occur because the medication has actually restored particular nerve cells to a state of normal functioning. When this takes place, normal brain function is restored and the experience generally does not feel like a "drug effect." In fact, most people report that they begin to "feel like themselves again." (For readers who are interested in a more detailed explanation of the effects of antidepressants, see Preston, O'Neal, and Talaga (1997).)

When brain functioning is restored, the most notable symptomatic changes are seen in the biological symptoms of depression (sleep, energy, etc.). Feelings of sadness, irritability, negative thinking, low self-esteem, and others of the "core symptoms" also respond; however, the most significant changes are seen in biologically based symptoms.

Unfortunately, antidepressants do not work rapidly. In almost every case in which the drugs eventually resolve the depression, it will require somewhere between two and four weeks of treatment to begin to see positive results. Furthermore, for these medications to work, they must be taken as prescribed and on a regular, daily basis. Much in the same way that antibiotics need some time to knock out an infection gradually, antidepressants require this amount of time to gradually restore the brain to a state of normal functioning.

Effectiveness of Antidepressants

The National Institute of Mental Health has determined that 80 percent or more of those suffering from depression can be successfully treated, and this also applies to those suffering from very serious cases of depression (NIMH: Fact Sheet 1990). The treatments to which the NIMH refer generally involve a combination of antidepressant medications and psychotherapy (we, too, strongly encourage this combined approach).

Currently there are more than twenty antidepressants on the market in the United States. These medications share some things in common, but each has particular effects (and side effects). In head-to-head comparisons between antidepressants, it has been found that all are equally effective. No one medication is superior in its effectiveness. However, these drugs differ considerably with regard to their side effects.

When being treated with antidepressants, it is essential to choose a medication with minimal or no side effects. Depressed people are already suffering a lot, and if they encounter significant side effects, many stop taking the medication, and thus do not experience symptom relief. So, although all antidepressants are equally effective, the reality is that those with fewer side effects (and thus better-tolerated) are much likelier to be taken as prescribed, and ultimately more successful.

The development of newer generation antidepressants that are significantly more user-friendly (i.e., many fewer side effects and judged to be much safer than earlier antidepressants) has been a major breakthrough of the past decade

Classes of Antidepressants

Not all antidepressants are alike. They all treat depression, but differ considerably in their chemical makeup and particular side effects. There are two broad classes of antidepressants that we will look at first: MAO-inhibitors and standard antidepressants.

MAO-Inhibitors

First developed in the 1950s, MAO-inhibitors are a specific class of antidepressants that work by inhibiting the action of a particular enzyme (monoamine-oxidase) in the brain. This enzyme metabolizes (or chemically degrades) the neurotransmitters serotonin, dopamine, and norepinephrine. Thus, MAO-inhibitors are able to block this process and thereby prevent the enzyme from lowering the level of these important brain chemicals. The particular action MAO-inhibitors use to normalize brain chemical levels is different than the action of standard antidepressants.

MAO-Inhibitors "No No" List

MAO-inhibitors are very effective antidepressants but, unfortunately, they may have some potentially dangerous drug-drug interactions (i.e., if combined with certain other medications, they can cause life-threatening reactions). Also, these drugs may have adverse interactions with a number of foods and alcoholic drinks (some of these interactions can be fatal). For this reason, when people are prescribed a MAO-inhibitor, they are advised about the potential risks and given a list of drugs and foods to avoid (see below). Because of these potential problems, MAO-inhibitors are not widely prescribed, although for some individuals they are the treatment of choice.

Foods to Avoid Completely

• Cheese (Philadelphia cream cheese, ricotta, and cottage cheese are OK.) • Chicken and beef liver • Sourdough bread • Canned yams • Yeast preparations (Avoid brewer's yeast, powdered and caked yeast as sold in health-food stores. Baker's yeast is OK.) • Fava or broad beans, Chinese pea pods, sauerkraut • Herring (pickled or kippered), smoked salmon, lox • Beer, sherry, ale, red wine, liqueurs, cognac, vermouth • Nonalcoholic beers and wines • Canned figs, banana peel • Protein extracts (found in some dried soups, soup cubes, and commercial gravies), tofu hot dogs • Some meat products: bologna, salami, pepperoni, Spam, some types of sausage, hot dogs, jerky, corned beef, liverwurst • Sour cream

Avoid Excessive Amounts of These Foods

• Yogurt, buttermilk • Ripe avocados and guacamole • Chocolate and/or caffeine • White wine and liquors • Fresh bacon or ham (Smoked bacon and ham are OK.) • Pate • Caviar • Peanuts

Medications to Avoid

• Stimulant drugs (amphetamines, Dexedrine, Benzedrine, methedrine, methylphenidate) • Diet pills • Cocaine, "Crack" cocaine • Cold preparations, including over-the-counter products that contain decongestants, e.g., Sudafed, Contac, etc. (Antihistamines and aspirin are OK.) • Nasal sprays (Saline and steroid nasal sprays are OK.) • Adrenaline (Make sure that your dentist knows you are taking MAO-inhibitors because many local anesthetics contain adrenaline.) • Tricyclic antidepressants • SSRI antidepressants • Buspirone (BuSpar) • Dextromethorphan • Levodopa • Demerol and other pain medications • Certain antihypertensive medications (for high blood pressure or migraine headaches)

Before taking any new medications (prescription or over-the-counter), be sure to talk to your physician or pharmacist about the medication's interactions with other drugs and food.

Standard Antidepressants

The second broad class of antidepressants is referred to as standard antidepressants (this list includes all *non*-MAO-inhibitor antidepressants). This group is comprised of the earliest generation of antidepressants (most were developed in the 1950s and 1960s) called *tricyclic antidepressants* and a number of newer agents commonly referred to as *second generation antidepressants* (developed in the late 1980s and in the 1990s). The currently available antidepressants are listed in table 5.1, along with additional information about typical doses and side effects.

Note: Part II, The Consumer's Guide to Psychiatric Drugs, provides detailed information about each psychiatric medication.

The standard antidepressants differ from each other in two ways. First, each has its own particular side effect profile. Second, each has a somewhat different effect on the various key neurotransmitters, serotonin, dopamine, and norepinephrine. As can be seen in table 5.1 some of these medications specifically target serotonin (5-HT) nerve cells (e.g., Prozac, Paxil). These antidepressants often referred to as SSRIs (selective serotonin reuptake inhibitors.) The term "reuptake" refers to the reabsorption of the neurotransmitter by the neuron that originally produced it.

Other standard antidepressants focus their actions exclusively on norepinephrine (NE) nerve cells (e.g., Norpramin, Ludiomil). Still others have an impact on two groups of nerve cells (e.g., Wellbutrin focuses on NE and dopamine (DA), and Remeron focuses on NE and 5-HT).

How do these actions on the activities of various nerve cells relate to the treatment of depression and the choice of medications? The research to date indicates that some people with depression suffer from a malfunction primarily in the serotonin system in the brain, while others' depression may be traceable to a disorder in norepinephrine system. Furthermore, some depressed people may have biological disturbances in their dopamine system, or combined disturbances in any of the three nerve cell systems. This is an important point, because there are those who are treated initially with an antidepressant that targets serotonin, and who exhibit either no response or only a partial response. If this occurs, it is important to know that it absolutely does not mean that antidepressants in general will be ineffective. Many of these patients will be switched to another class of antidepressants (e.g.,

Table 5.1 Antidepressants At a Glance

ANTIDEPRESSANT Names		Usual Daily		Weight		Selective Action On Neurotransmitters[1]	
Generic	Brand	Dosage Range	Sedation	Gain	ACH[2]	NE	5-HT
imipramine	Tofranil	150–300 mg	mid	mid	mid	mid	mid
desipramine	Norpramin	150–300 mg	low	low	low	high	none
amitriptyline	Elavil	150–300 mg	high	high	high	low	high
nortriptyline	Aventyl, Pamelor	75–125 mg	mid	low	mid	mid	mid
protriptyline	Vivactil	15–40 mg	mid	low	mid	high	low
trimipramine	Surmontil	100–300 mg	high	high	mid	mid	mid
doxepin	Sinequan, Adapin	150–300 mg	high	high	high	mid	mid
maprotiline	Ludiomil	150–225 mg	high	mid	mid	mid	none
amoxapine	Asendin	150–400 mg	mid	low	low	high	low
trazodone	Desyrel	150–400 mg	mid	low	none	none	high
fluoxetine	Prozac	20–80 mg	low	none	none	none	high
bupropion-S.R.	Wellbutrin-S.R.	150–300 mg	low	none	none	mid	none
bupropion	Wellbutrin	150–400 mg	low	none	none	mid	none
sertraline	Zoloft	50–200 mg	low	none	none	none	high
paroxetine	Paxil	20–50 mg	low	none	low	none	high
venlafaxine-X.R.	Effexor-X.R.	75–300 mg	low	none	none	mid	mid
venlafaxine	Effexor	75–375 mg	low	none	none	mid	mid
nefazodone	Serzone	100–500 mg	mid	none	none	low	high
fluvoxamine	Luvox	50–300 mg	low	none	low	none	high
mirtazapine	Remeron	15–45 mg	mid	high	mid	mid	mid
MAO-INHIBITORS							
phenelzine	Nardil	30–90 mg	low	mid	none	mid	mid
tranylcypromine	Parnate	20–60 mg	low	low	none	mid	mid

[1] Action on neurotransmitters. NE: Norepinephrine. 5-HT: Serotonin.

[2] ACH: Anticholinergic effects: dry mouth, constipation, blurry vision, urinary hesitation.

one targeting norepinephrine) and then go on to have a very good response.

Here is the problem: It is often difficult for doctors to know which group of antidepressants ultimately will prove effective. There are some guidelines outlined below that can aid the physician in choosing a medication, but often the choice must be made on a trial and error basis, starting treatment with one medication and being prepared to switch to another should the patient fail to show a good response.

What to Expect from Medication Treatment

It is very important for people starting treatment, to be well informed regarding the effects of the medication and, in particular, what to expect.

Choosing an Antidepressant

Once the diagnosis and the decision to use antidepressant medications have been made, the physician will recommend a particular medication. Since the newer generation antidepressants are much better in terms of their side-effect profiles, typically, Prozac, Paxil, Zoloft, or Wellbutrin is chosen as a first-line medication.

First-Line Choices

Several factors influence the particular choice of a first-line medication. Of course these factors vary considerably from one physician to another; however, several common guidelines that may influence this decision are listed below:

- Generally, if there have been previous depressive episodes and a particular medication was used successfully, the doctor will recommend using that same medication again.

- Side-effect considerations: the physician will take careful note of each patient's medical history, age, gender, and other factors and, based on this information, will choose a medication that seems best-suited to the particular patient, with regard to its side effects. For example, if the patient is overweight, the doctor will be careful not to choose a medication that typically has weight gain as a side effect. Or, if the patient is experiencing significant fatigue and daytime drowsiness, the doctor is likely to choose an antidepressant that has minimal or no sedating side effects.

- A review of other medications currently taken by the patient will help the physician choose an antidepressant that is not likely to cause dangerous drug-drug interactions.

- The particular pattern of depressive symptoms can *sometimes* be a factor in medication choices. For example, people suffering from depression and Obsessive Compulsive Disorder (OCD) (see chapter 7) have been found to respond best to antidepressants that target serotonin (e.g., SSRIs like Prozac or Paxil); individuals who suffer from very severe, recurrent depressions have been shown to respond somewhat more favorably to drugs that have an impact on norepinephrine (e.g., Wellbutrin or Norpramin).

These are the primary factors influencing the initial choice of medication. Whether an individual continues to be treated with a specific antidepressant will depend on two factors: first, whether it is well tolerated (i.e., has no or minimal side effects), and second, how well the medication works to alleviate depressive symptoms.

Antidepressant Doses

For any antidepressant medication to be effective, it must be taken at an adequate dose. One of the more common reasons that people fail to respond to antidepressant treatment is because of inadequate dosages. (This may be caused either by patients taking the medication on an irregular basis or by the medication having been prescribed at a subtherapeutic dose.) To work properly, it is essential that these medications be taken on a regular, daily basis, as prescribed.

Initially, many of the antidepressants are prescribed at a low dose, which is taken for a few days to see if it is well tolerated, and then the dosage is increased gradually to a level that is likely to be effective. Some of the newer medications (e.g., Prozac, Zoloft, Paxil, or Wellbutrin, SR) may be started at the full dosage level. The precise dosage for any individual patient will depend on a number of factors that must be determined by the treating physician. Table 5.1 "Antidepressants at a Glance" on page 65 does list common therapeutic dosage ranges for adults ages sixteen to sixty.

Note: Doses for people over the age of sixty generally are lower.

Phases of Treatment

Recently, several psychiatric groups have made specific recommendations regarding the treatment of depression. The following sections outline the generally agreed-upon treatment guidelines, and focus on three specific phases of medical treatment.

Phase One: Acute Treatment: This phase begins with the first dose of an antidepressant and continues until most or all of the depressive symptoms have disappeared. As noted earlier, in most cases (with all antidepressants) it is necessary to take the medication each day as directed, and typically it will take from two to four weeks of treatment before the first signs of improvement are noted. For those suffering from depression, this waiting period often seems incredibly long, but it is absolutely necessary. The antidepressant must have a continuous effect on the malfunctioning nerve cells for this length of time in order to begin the process of normalizing brain functioning. If the correct medication has been selected and it is taken as prescribed, then it is likely that the first signs of improvement will be noticed some time in this two-to-four week period.

Generally, the first signs of improvement include the following: better quality sleep, decreased fatigue, decreased agitation, and a better sense of emotional control (i.e., patients will still feel emotions of sadness or anger, etc., but they often report an enhanced sense of control over these feelings). Other symptoms of depression usually take longer to respond. In successful treatments, many if not most depressive symptoms will be resolved within six to eight weeks after initiating treatment. In other cases, the response may not be as positive, and other measures must be used to increase a positive response.

The acute phase of treatment ends when the person is no longer suffering from the major symptoms of depression. Many people when they begin to feel "normal" again, naturally assume that they can stop taking the antidepressant at this time.

Caution: Despite the fact that they *feel* fully recovered, a very large percentage of patients will relapse quickly if they stop taking antidepressants at this time. It is strongly advised that additional time be spent continuing the medication.

Phase Two: Continuation Treatment: This phase of treatment begins where the acute phase leaves off. The general guideline is for the patient to continue taking the antidepressant *at the same dosage as during phase one* for a minimum of six months. This has been shown to play an important role in preventing acute relapse. After this additional six months of treatment, many people can then discontinue treatment and they will not have a sudden relapse. It must be noted, however, as mentioned earlier, that in many instances depression will reoccur. This can take place several years after the first episode. Thus, treatment with antidepressants can be effective in resolving the current episode, and an extra six months of treatment often prevents an acute (or sudden) return of depressive symptoms. It will not, however, provide long-lasting protection from future episodes. (Longer-term relapse prevention is discussed below in the section on phase three.)

Phase Three: Maintenance Treatment: If someone has been treated successfully for a *first episode* of clinical depression, and has completed phase two, as a rule, the physician will recommend discontinuation of the medications. Typically, this will involve a gradual reduction of the dosage over a period of a few weeks. When this is completed, and assuming that depressive symptoms do not reappear, then treatment is considered ended. All patients who have gone through an episode of depression should be made aware that depression can recur, and be taught to watch for any signs of reemerging depressive symptoms. Should symptoms reoccur, it is important to see a therapist or physician as soon as possible, because rapid treatment may prevent another full-blown episode.

If the depressive episode being treated is a second, third, or subsequent one, many (if not most) psychiatrists will recommend ongoing antidepressant treatment (possibly indefinitely) because long-term treatment has proven quite effective in preventing relapse. Many people, however, are reluctant to consider long-term medication use, although it has been clearly established that this can be a highly effective approach to relapse prevention. In cases of recurring depression, it is not uncommon for later episodes to become even more severe and difficult to treat, thus the prevention of additional episodes becomes crucial. Furthermore, to date there is little evidence to suggest that very long-term treatment is dangerous. A large number of patients have been treated with antidepressants continuously for more than two decades without any evidence of harmful effects to their major organ systems. Additionally, the alternative to long-term treatment (uncontrolled, and increasingly severe episodes) can carry grave consequences.

Side Effects

All medications, prescription or over-the counter, have side effects. It is important for patients to know about their particular prescription and its unique side-effect profile. Many people treated with antidepressants notice no side effects at all. For those who do encounter side effects, generally, the effects are minimal and not dangerous. This is especially the case with the newer generation of antidepressants. Table 5.1 provides a quick look at some common side effects of antidepressants and Part II of this book, the Drug Guide, can help you to locate your particular antidepressant and review a fairly complete list of possible side effects.

In almost all cases, side effects can be managed (either by a dosage adjustment or by a switch to another medication). Thus, it is very important to notify your treating therapist or physician if you encounter any significant side-effect problems. Unfortunately, many depressed people who encounter side effects simply stop taking the medication, and continue to suffer.

Note: Solutions to side-effect problems can almost always be found.

Precautions and Contraindications

Antidepressant medications, especially the newer generation drugs, have been found to be very safe. However, as with all medical treatments, some precautions are in order. First, it is important to know that several groups of people should either not take antidepressants or do so only under careful medical observation. These groups include pregnant women, people with seizure disorders, people with known allergies to antidepressants, people with narrow angle glaucoma, and those who have recently sustained a heart attack.

There are some patients with these disorders or conditions who may be treated with antidepressants, but they must be monitored very carefully.

Caution: If antidepressants are taken at very high doses (for example, in an intentional or accidental overdose), the consequences can be grave. The newer antidepressants, fortunately, are much safer in this regard, but they can present serious medical complications if taken in inappropriately high doses. Thus, it is extremely important to take medications only as prescribed, and if you or a loved one has ingested an excessive amount of an antidepressant, consider it a medical emergency and seek medical treatment immediately.

It is also important not to drink a great deal of alcohol while taking antidepressants. Typically, consuming one drink is not dangerous. However, ingesting a moderate-to-heavy amount of alcohol can be very risky indeed, and is extremely ill-advised.

Finally, it is important to know that there are some potentially dangerous drug-drug interactions, not only with MAO-inhibitors, but also with standard antidepressants. A list of the more common potential drug-drug interactions can be found for each specific medication in Part II. Also, be sure to discuss the safety of combining antidepressants with any prescription or over-the-counter drugs with your physician or pharmacist.

Are Antidepressants Addictive or Habit-Forming?

The question about addiction is a common one and it is completely understandable. The answer is that *antidepressants are absolutely not addictive*. There is no evidence either from animal or human studies or from clinical findings that antidepressants are addictive or habit-forming. However, it must be emphasized that some people are treated for depression with *other classes of drugs* that *can* be habit-forming. These medications are not antidepressants, rather they are stimulants (e.g., Dexedrine) or minor tranquilizers (e.g., Valium). There are appropriate medical uses of stimulants and tranquilizers and in some isolated cases they may be used appropriately as a part of treatment for depression. In this chapter, however, the focus is exclusively on the use of antidepressants, and these medications are neither addictive nor habit-forming.

Is Long-Term Use of Antidepressants Safe?

Because many people will be treated with antidepressants for a prolonged period of time, the question of the safety of long-term use is important. There are individuals who have been treated continuously for more than two decades with the early generation antidepressants (the tricyclic antidepressants such as imipramine and nortriptyline), without demonstrating any evidence of adverse impact on their major organ systems. These drugs appear to be quite safe for very long-term use. The newer medications have not been available long enough to be certain about their long-term effect on the human body (e.g., there are people who have been treated with Prozac and some of the other newer antidepressants for more than ten years, but not for longer periods of time). At this time, there are no indications of adverse effects in those individuals. However, in the absence of data collected over a period of many years, the question of safety is difficult to determine in an absolute way.

When addressing the issue of long-term safety, one very important question is, "What are the risks of not using the medication?" For depression, this can be answered with some assurance. The lifetime mortality rate for death by suicide in people with recurrent depression is somewhere between 12 and 15 percent. Furthermore, if the disorder goes untreated, depression has been associated with significantly higher rates of physical illness.

Finally, the toll taken on the quality of an individual's life when depression is not treated must be addressed. Thus, based on available data, it seems clear that the decision *not to treat* results in significant risk while long-term medication treatment appears to be accompanied by little risk to physical health.

What if the First Treatment Is Not Successful?

In the medical treatment of most cases of clinical depression, the hoped-for effect will be some noticeable symptom reduction within the first two to four weeks. When this occurs, it is generally the case that additional improvement will be seen over the next few weeks. However, two classes of difficulties may arise: partial response to the medication or no response at all.

The first difficulty occurs when the patient demonstrates only a partial response by week four. Before increasing the dosage or prescribing another medication, it must first be determined that:

- The diagnosis of depression is correct

- The patient is, in fact, taking the medication as prescribed

- There is no ongoing alcohol or other substance abuse

Once these issues have been evaluated, then the standard approach is to increase the dose of the antidepressant (always with careful monitoring to be sure that significant side effects do not emerge). It is not unusual that an increase in dose will yield good results. Should the first dose adjustment not be successful, the dose can continue to be increased, as long as side effect problems do not interfere. The doctor may also request a blood test to determine if the medication is reaching high enough levels in the person's bloodstream.

Should these attempts fail to result in significant improvement, then two standard strategies are often employed. One high-yield approach is to add a second medicine to the one already being taken. This approach is referred to as augmentation. Common augmentation choices include the addition of lithium or thyroid hormone to the antidepressant, or the addition of an antidepressant from another class of antidepressants (for example adding Wellbutrin, a NE antidepressant, to Prozac, which is an SSRI). Drug augmentation is very effective in about 50 percent of those who have exhibited only marginal responses to the initial antidepressant.

The second kind of difficulty occurs when the initial drug produces no symptom reduction during the first four to six weeks, despite dosage increases. In such cases, a common strategy is to stop the antidepressant, and start treatment anew with a different medication; generally from another class (for example, switching from an SSRI like Zoloft to a medication that targets NE like Norpramin).

Medication adjustments and augmentation strategies can be complex and very individualized, and thus it is beyond the scope of this book to discuss all of the possibilities here. However, it is important for those who do not experience a good response to their first medication to know that many options exist. They should not give up and conclude, "Antidepressants do not work for me." The vast majority of people with clinical depression do respond, and they respond well—once the right medication or combination of medications is found.

Ineffective and Dangerous Treatments for Clinical Depression

One very common mistake made in the treatment of clinical depression is the use of antianxiety medications (also referred to as minor tranquilizers). Many people who suffer from depression also experience anxiety and agitation. For this reason they are sometimes misdiagnosed, assumed to have an anxiety disorder or some form of generic "stress," and they are prescribed tranquilizers. This is often a significant mistake. As a rule, minor tranquilizers are not effective for treating depression, and, in fact, they often worsen depression over time. When anxiety is present in the context of major depression, antidepressant medications almost always succeed in alleviating the anxiety and/or agitation, as well as the depression.

In the 1950s and 1960s physicians tried the use of stimulants to treat depression. Not only were these attempts unsuccessful, in many cases there were disastrous consequences (including drug addiction). Stimulants include drugs such as Dexedrine and street drugs such as amphetamines and cocaine. *Antidepressants are not stimulants.* They are chemically different and operate in quite different ways than stimulants do. Most notably, antidepressants are not addictive while stimulants can be and usually are. On rare occasions stimulants may be used in cases of depression, but, generally, they are not currently considered a viable treatment.

Various herbal and so-called "natural" treatments have been recommended for treating depression. Some of these include the use of tyrosine, tryptophan, or ginseng. These products do not appear to be effective for treating major depression. The remedy receiving the most media attention lately has been an extract from the flower, *St. John's Wort.* The studies available at this time do offer some promise for the use of this product in the treatment of mild depression. However, the data to date are still limited, and people suffering from moderate-to-severe depression should discuss the use of this agent with their doctor.

Diet and Depression

Finally, what about diet? It is clear that the basic neurotransmitters implicated in depression are manufactured in the brain, and rely on some essential amino acids (derived through diet) as their chemical building blocks. Consequently, it is no surprise that there has been a lot of speculation about the role of diet in emotional illness (especially depression). It is also true that many, if not most, people in the throes of depression do not practice good health habits (they tend to avoid exercise, drink too much alcohol, smoke too much, and eat a poor diet). Certainly, establishing healthy habits (including a good diet) is important, especially when recovering from depression. However, research to date has *failed* to demonstrate that dietary approaches for treating clinical depression are successful.

Nonmedical Treatments for Depression

As noted earlier, psychotherapy is the primary nonmedical treatment for depression, with a well documented track record of effectiveness. Beyond this there are a few other nonmedical approaches worth noting. At the top of the list is exercise. Regular strenuous exercise has clearly been shown to improve the quality of sleep. There is also mounting evidence that regular exercise increases the amount of serotonin in the brain. For these reasons, it has proved to be an important adjunct in the treatment of depression.

Light Therapy

Light therapy is another nonmedical approach. In the past decade a great deal was learned about the need for daylight. When one's exposure to daylight is inadequate, this often has a dramatic effect on sleep patterns, hormone levels, and mood. This effect is most pronounced in those who suffer from what is now called Seasonal Affective Disorder (SAD).

Such people have a strong tendency to become quite depressed each year during the winter months. Worldwide, the incidence of SAD has been found to be consistently higher in geographic locations farther away from the Equator and closer to the poles. For instance, although the incidence of those people in

Florida who experience SAD is about 1.5 percent, the incidence in New England is about 9.5 percent (Rosenthal 1994). After years of careful study, it has been determined that the decrease in exposure to bright light is the culprit. So it should come as no surprise that SAD is also common in those who work night shifts (about 20 percent of working adults in the United States), who sleep during the day, and thus get little exposure to bright light.

The current theory holds that, like most animals, humans evolved and developed biological systems that respond to and are "in synch" with the environment. One aspect of the environment is the amount of daily light exposure. Light therapy has been found to be very effective for patients with SAD. This involves daily exposure to a source of bright light (either by way of commercially available light boxes, or by making a point of going outside each day, and receiving a certain amount of exposure to sunlight).

The details of light therapy treatment for SAD are beyond the scope of this book, however, the interested reader is referred to Dr. Rosenthal's excellent book (1994).

Caution: For those with a history of bipolar (manic-depressive) illness, light therapy should be done only under medical supervision, because it can, at times, cause such an individual to shift into a manic state.

Dysthymia

As described above, episodes of major depression are often extremely intense, and, if not treated, typically last for a number of months. In addition to these kinds of episodic depressions, there are also those who suffer from a very long-lasting type of low-grade depression, referred to as dysthymia. It is believed that this disorder affects about 6 percent of the population (Kessler et al. 1994). Typically, it begins in childhood or adolescence and continues for many, many years (often for a lifetime). With dysthymia, the depression does not reach the depths of that seen in major depression, and most dysthymic people continue to function (i.e., they can carry out the tasks of daily life). However, their lives are burdened by an almost constant low-grade depression. This usually manifests in the following symptoms: feelings of inadequacy or low self-esteem, persistent lack of enthusiasm, fatigue, no zest for life, irritability, and a strong tendency for negative, pessimistic thinking.

People with dysthymia can be treated by psychotherapy, and some recent studies have shown that a number of persons with dysthymia also respond to antidepressant medications. The response rate to medication treatments is about 55 percent (Stewart et al. 1992; Akiskal and Weise 1992). This is certainly less than the response rates seen when treating major depression, but for those who do have a good response, medication treatment can be a godsend.

When medication treatments are successful for people with dysthymia, these patients often make comments like, "I have never felt this good in my entire life." This kind of very positive result has led many investigators to conclude that probably some forms of dysthymia are caused by a chronic neurobiological malfunction. What remains unclear, assuming that patients have demonstrated a good response to antidepressants, is—how long must they be treated?

One research finding worth noting is that the older generation tricyclic medications are not especially effective in treating dysthymia. Most of the older generation drugs primarily target norepinephrine. More recent findings suggest that the classes of medications that may be most effective for treating dysthymia are either MAO-inhibitors or SSRIs (Davidson 1997).

Premenstrual Dysphoria

About 75 percent of all women notice some changes in their emotions when they are premenstrual. For most, the changes are slight. However, it has been estimated that about 5 percent of women (APA 1994a, 716) experience very intense mood symptoms during this part of their menstrual cycle, referred to as *premenstrual dysphoria*. The emotional changes can include depression, anxiety, and/or irritability. During the past five years many psychiatric specialists have noted that the serotonin antidepressants (SSRIs) appear to be effective in reducing these mood symptoms (and are more effective in accomplishing this than other classes of antidepressants). The emotional brain is packed with estrogen-sensitive receptors, and it makes sense that significant fluctuations in female hormones (especially estrogen) may destabilize the chemical functioning in the limbic system.

There are two main strategies for using SSRIs to treat premenstrual mood changes. Treatment in which the woman takes antidepressants continuously (i.e., not just premenstrually) is the most common. The second, still somewhat experimental strategy, is sometimes effective for those women who are depressed only for the few days they are premenstrual, i.e., they do not experience intense mood changes any other time of the month. This approach involves using SSRIs only on those days during which the woman experiences symptoms.

It should be noted that exercise, exposure to bright light, and some dietary changes also may play an important role in the treatment of premenstrual dysphoria.

Atypical Depression

It has been estimated that between 15 and 20 percent of people experiencing clinical depression, suffer from a particular subtype of major depression called *Atypical Depression* (atypical meaning not typical) (Davidson 1997). The symptoms of atypical depression include the following: severe fatigue, appetite *increase* and weight *gain*, and excessive sleeping (unlike more typical depressions where insomnia is a problem, with atypical depression there is a strong need to sleep a lot, e.g., 10–14 hours a day). Also, many people suffering from atypical depression are prone to anxiety and sometimes to panic attacks (see chapter 7).

One reason for listing this disorder separately is that it may have a specific underlying neurochemical cause, and thus respond best to a specific class of antidepressants. In fact, it has been shown that people with atypical depression respond best to treatment with MAO-inhibitors. Some of these people also respond well to a second class of antidepressants, the SSRIs. Antidepressants that target norepinephrine (e.g., the tricyclics) have not been found to be as effective as the MAO-inhibitors or the SSRIs.

Psychotic Depression

Some types of major depression can become so severe that there is a significant breakdown of the personality. When this occurs, patients begin to suffer from what are known as psychotic symptoms. The most common psychotic symptoms seen in severe major depression include the following:

- Delusions (extremely unrealistic and even bizarre beliefs, e.g., "I am the devil" . . . "I am dead" . . . "My internal organs are rotten." Such ideas are easily recognized as being clearly out of touch with reality.)

- Hallucinations (such as hearing voices)

- Gross disorganization and confusion

- Extreme neglect of hygiene

- Refusal to eat (which can become life threatening)

- Profoundly impaired judgment (Such people may not be able to appreciate the seriousness of their condition and may refuse to cooperate with treatment.)

It is also important to know that during periods of psychotic depression, *the suicide risk is very high.* In every instance of psychotic depression, immediate treatment should be sought.

Psychotherapy alone is rarely helpful for those in the midst of a psychotic depression. Medical treatment is always warranted, which may include psychiatric hospitalization. Two medical treatments have proved to be effective with psychotic depression. The first is the combined use of antidepressants *and* antipsychotic medications. Either class of medication alone is not very effective. It is clear that appropriate treatment must include both (see also chapter 8).

Electro-Convulsive Therapy (ECT)

The second-line treatment is ECT (electro-convulsive therapy), commonly referred to as "shock therapy." Electro-convulsive therapy was first developed in the late 1930s. When initially employed it was, unfortunately, inappropriately used to treat a wide variety of mental illnesses. The early procedures were crude and some resulted in dangerous consequences for patients. The treatment took on an ominous appearance, especially as it was depicted in the media. However, ECT was found to be tremendously effective for a particular subgroup of psychiatric patients: those suffering from extremely severe depression, especially psychotic depression.

Fortunately, significant changes took place in the past two decades. The technique was refined and now can be conducted in a very safe and effective manner. Today, ECT is administered with the patient under a general anesthesia, and monitored by a team of physicians and nurses. In the 1990s, ECT is considered a safe treatment with few, if any, lasting side effects. It is especially effective for treating psychotic depression; however, ECT is almost always accompanied by psychiatric medication treatment.

Note: As effective as ECT is for initial treatment of severe depression, without ongoing medication treatment, relapses are common.

Bipolar Disorders

Introduction

In the most general sense, bipolar disorder, which is also known as manic depression, is characterized by wide swings in mood that alternate between mania and depression. These two emotional states can be viewed as opposite ends, or "poles," of a continuum, hence the term *bipolar* (*bi* is the Latin term for two). During an episode of mania a person's mood is abnormally elevated or euphoric. The depression associated with bipolar disorder can be equal in severity to major depression (see chapter 5 for a detailed discussion of major depression) and is recognized by feelings of intense sadness and hopelessness. Actually, there are several different types of bipolar disorder; however, central to all types are the swings between an elevated mood and a depressed mood.

On average, one percent of the U.S. adult population is afflicted with bipolar disorder (American Psychiatric Association 1994b). It often first appears in adolescence or early adulthood and is considered a long-term illness, characterized by patterns of multiple episodes. The average number of episodes of either mania or depression in a lifetime is approximately ten. The interval between episodes, called cycles, can vary from person to person. It is not uncommon for five or more years to pass between the first and second episode. However, over a lifetime, the periods between subsequent episodes become shorter in duration. The average episode lasts between four and twelve months, manic phases being somewhat shorter (Judd, Braff, Britton, et al. 1991). It is important to emphasize that in spite of the general estimates of cycling frequency and length, described above, bipolar disorder is extremely variable in its course.

There are effective treatments for bipolar disorder; however, it is important to recognize that the consequences of this disease can be devastating. There are significant negative effects on marital and family relationships, on occupational or school functioning, and on quality of life. Compared to the general population, divorce rates are two to three times higher and job performance is twice as likely to be impaired. Substance abuse, recklessness, and inflicting harm on oneself or others are commonly associated with bipolar disorder. There is a high risk of suicide. At least 15 to 20 percent of those with bipolar disorder will attempt suicide (American Psychiatric Association 1994b).

For the majority of people with the disorder, the symptoms of bipolar disorder can be treated effectively. However, for about 20 to 30 percent, the course of their illness will be more difficult. For some people core symptoms will not respond adequately to treatment. Others may experience some degree of mood swings on a chronic basis even if their most intense symptoms have been relieved (Keller, Lavori, Coryell, et al. 1993; American Psychiatric Association 1994b; Solomon, Keitner, Miller, et al. 1995; Goldberg, Harrow, and Grossman 1995; Evans, Byerly, and Greer 1995; Calabrese, Fatemi, Kujawa, et al. 1996; Keck and MeElroy 1996).

Making the Diagnosis

As with any psychological or medical diagnosis, having a clear understanding of the core symptoms is essential. *Mania* is considered to be an abnormally elevated mood that persists for one week or more. This state is often described as a "natural high" and someone who is manic may deny that this mood is abnormal and will resist attempts at help or treatment. Even though mania can exist in mild, moderate, or severe forms, generally, it causes significant impairment in daily functioning.

In addition to the elevated mood, it is very important that the associated behaviors be recognized. These behaviors, such as spending sprees and inappropriate sexual activity, can cause significant difficulty and distress in the lives of all involved. Hospitalization is often required during a manic episode to ensure the safety of the individual and to start treatment that would otherwise not be adhered to or refused.

At the most extreme, during a manic episode a person can suffer from psychotic symptoms such as hallucinations (hearing voices or seeing images that do not exist in reality) or delusions (bizarre and unrealistic beliefs). These psychotic symptoms clearly indicate a loss of contact with reality. There is often an observable disorganization in speech, and an inability to carry out normal daily activities, such as eating or bathing.

Hypomania

Hypomania is another important term to understand. A *hypomanic episode* differs from a manic episode in that social or occupational functioning is not appreciably impaired. As in mania, the mood is abnormally elevated, and many of the associated behaviors are present. However, hypomania does not involve psychotic symptoms and most daily functioning is maintained. Hospitalization is not required to treat a hypomanic episode.

In both mania and hypomania there can be a strong desire on the part of the individual to continue in this state. Patients often say that they are at their most creative or productive when in a manic or hypomanic state. There may be a tendency to achieve this "high" and maintain it. This often translates into a refusal to seek help or adhere to treatment that has been prescribed previously.

Core Symptoms of Mania

- Excessive euphoric or high feelings

- Extreme irritability

- Distractibility

- Unrealistic and inflated beliefs in one's abilities—this is called *grandiosity*

- Dramatic mannerisms

- Racing thoughts, called *flight of ideas*

- Loud, pressured, and rapid speech—difficult to interrupt and subject to changing topics, often unrelated
- Increased energy, activity, restlessness
- Decreased need for sleep
- Increased sex drive—provocative behavior, can be aggressive or promiscuous
- Poor judgment
- Abuse of substances, particularly stimulants and alcohol
- Spending sprees

Note that the physiological symptoms of depression, as well as the core symptoms of depression, both outlined below, are also characteristic of the *depressed phase* of bipolar disorder.

Core Symptoms of Depression

- Mood of sadness, despair, emptiness
- Anhedonia (loss of ability to experience pleasure)
- Low self-esteem
- Apathy, low motivation, and social withdrawal
- Excessive emotional sensitivity
- Negative, pessimistic thinking
- Irritability
- Suicidal thoughts

Physiological Symptoms of Depression

- Appetite disturbance, either decreased or increased, with accompanying weight loss or gain
- Fatigue
- Decreased sex drive
- Restlessness, agitation, or psychomotor retardation
- Diurnal variations in mood—usually feeling worse in the morning
- Impaired concentration and forgetfulness

- Pronounced anhedonia—total loss of ability to experience pleasure
- Sleep disturbance—waking very early in the morning, frequently waking throughout the night, sleeping excessively

The Subtypes of Bipolar Disorder

There are three common subtypes of bipolar disorder: Bipolar I, Bipolar II, and Cyclothymia. Although a full diagnostic discussion is beyond the scope of this book, it is worth noting that there can be accompanying features to a bipolar diagnosis. For instance, sometimes bipolar disorder is associated with a seasonal pattern or shortly after childbirth.

Bipolar I

The diagnosis of *Bipolar I* is generally made when there has been at least one major depressive episode and at least one episode of mania. The diagnosis also may be made based on the presence of a single manic episode, with no past depressive episodes. This diagnosis comes closest to the historical concept of classic bipolar disorder. The bipolar I subtype is equally common in women and men. Sometimes there can be feelings of mania and depression concurrently within the same twenty-four-hour period. If such a pattern persists, this is called the *mixed type* of Bipolar I disorder.

Bipolar II

Bipolar II is diagnosed when there has been at least one episode of major depression and at least one episode of hypomania. Because hypomanic symptoms may be more subtle than mania, this diagnosis is sometimes difficult to establish. Hypomania is not always experienced as euphoria, rather some people will describe "being extremely irritable" or "having a low frustration tolerance." More women than men have Bipolar II disorder (American Psychiatric Association 1994b).

For both Bipolar I and II, an especially difficult to treat cycling pattern may develop, called *rapid cycling*. This means that a person has four or more episodes of depression, or mania, or hypomania, in a twelve-month period. Between 10 and 20 percent of people with bipolar disorder are rapid cyclers. More women than men experience rapid cycling (American Psychiatric Association 1994b).

Cyclothymia

Cyclothymia involves a long-term cyclic pattern of both hypomanic and depressive symptoms. The depressive symptoms are not severe enough nor long enough in duration to be considered a major depression.

Other Diagnostic Issues

Mania may occur as a consequence of certain medical conditions, or it may be induced by medication treatment or recreational drugs. The following sections show examples of each. Note that these causes of mania do not contribute to large numbers of cases of bipolar disorder.

Depression also can be caused by various medical conditions. These are discussed in detail in chapter 5.

Medical Conditions Causally Associated with Mania

- Injury or trauma to the brain, e.g., stroke
- Hyperthyroidism
- Infections such as encephalitis
- Seizure disorders
- Brain tumors

Drugs that Can Induce Mania

- Stimulants, e.g., cocaine or amphetamines
- Certain antidepressants, notably tricyclics
- Some medications used to lower blood pressure
- Steroid antiinflammatory medications in higher doses, such as prednisone
- Anticholinergic medications, such as benztropine
- Thyroid hormones, such as levothyroxine

Is a Medical or Psychiatric Exam Necessary?

Evaluation by a medical doctor, or psychiatrist, and sometimes both, is often necessary. Medical causes of the symptoms may need to be identified and treated. If medications are suspected, they will have to be changed and the underlying medical condition stabilized. This is especially true if the first episode of mania emerges in someone forty years of age or older (American Psychiatric Association 1994b). Most mood stabilizing medications used to treat bipolar disorder necessitate laboratory measurements that require a physician's monitoring.

Bipolar Disorder and the Brain

Bipolar disorder was first described in the early 1920s and much research is still needed to yield a more complete understanding of what occurs in the brain during manic or depressed states. Proposed theories focus primarily on biological and genetic causes, and less on environmental influences, although the latter have great importance. Many of the same neurotransmitter systems implicated in depression and anxiety, i.e., serotonin, norepinephrine, dopamine and GABA (gamma-amino butyric acid) are assumed to be dysregulated in bipolar disorder, most likely in some combination. However, the manner in which these neurotransmitter systems are dysregulated varies between disorders. The term dysregulated does not mean that something is broken or lacking in the brain. Rather, it means that these systems are working in a less than optimal way.

Because bipolar disorder is characterized by its cyclic nature, there have been attempts to determine whether mania and depression can be explained by an interruption in normal biological rhythms. In particular, the circadian cycle may be disrupted and become unpredictable (American Psychiatric Association 1994b).

Because some of the medications used to treat bipolar disorder are anticonvulsants, researchers have looked for a link between the brain activity patterns of people with seizure disorders and compared them to people with bipolar disorder (Ballenger and Post 1980). The particular mechanism in question is called *kindling*. This is a process in which the brain becomes progressively sensitive to various stimuli, both normal and stressful. Over time, the sensitization increases to a point where the brain spontaneously begins to show abnormal activity, even when there are no stressful triggering events. Although such a connection makes intuitive sense, this area of research has not yet provided any conclusive evidence.

Research Limits

Research efforts are extensive in the area of bipolar disorder. However, there are certain limits that impede progress. For instance, carrying out studies in those who are acutely manic is difficult due to their hyperactivity and tendency to be uncooperative. Sometimes, genetic studies are carried out initially with just a small group of subjects. When these same studies are repeated with a larger number of people, the original conclusions are not supported.

There is fairly strong evidence that, in some cases, bipolar disorder runs in families. Currently, researchers have not identified a particular genetic means of transmission, but it is known that the occurrence of bipolar disorder increases if close relatives also have the disorder. Drawing any conclusions about a genetic predisposition must be done cautiously since the role of environmental factors in the disorder is also thought to be of major importance (American Psychiatric Association 1994b; Tsuang and Faraone 1990; Baron et al. 1987). In sum, it is thought that there is a strong inherited vulnerability for bipolar disorder. However, the degree of this vulnerability is not uniform and varies greatly from person to person.

Treatments for Bipolar Disorder

Bipolar disorder is predominantly treated with medication. Two other components of treatment are also extremely important. The first is education and adjustment of lifestyle to minimize future episodes. Family members and significant others who participate in this education and modification of lifestyle can greatly help a person deal effectively with bipolar disorder.

Psychotherapy also has a place in the treatment of bipolar disorder. It is most effective when provided in a supportive manner and aimed at helping the clients to recognize the impact that the symptoms of bipolar disorder have on their lives. This type of therapy helps people to gain insight into their behavior and learn how to avoid painful repetitions.

When interviewing a therapist be sure to look for someone who is skilled in treating bipolar disorder. It is also important that the therapist have an established relationship with a psychiatrist, so that medications can be managed successfully and compliance enhanced. In practice, most primary care physicians will refer a person with bipolar disorder to a psychiatrist, because of the specialized care required. We agree with this practice and recommend that, in most cases, bipolar disorder should be treated by a psychiatrist rather than a primary care provider.

Education and Lifestyle Adjustment

Education will be most effective when provided on an ongoing basis. The ability for someone who is manic to retain information may be compromised. Sharing factual information repeatedly over time in different ways is more effective than providing the information only one time. Informed people will also be more confident in their ability to manage their lives. With that confidence comes the ability to implement the recommended lifestyle changes.

The Key Elements of Education and Lifestyle Factors

- Learn as much as you can about bipolar disorder.
- Learn as much as you can about your medications.
- Adhere to prescribed treatment—not doing so will lead to relapse.
- Be patient with your treatment regimen—it may take some time for the proper medications or dosages to be found.
- Accept that sometimes hospitalization may be necessary if symptoms are particularly severe.
- Report symptoms early so that treatment can be started or changed as soon as possible.
- Establish regular sleeping and eating cycles—keep a written record if necessary to help establish a consistent daily schedule.
- Keep an accurate, chronological record of when episodes occur, how severe they are, what might have triggered them, and how long they last.

- Recognize that stressful life events can trigger manic or depressed episodes.
- Ask for feedback from others about how you are doing.
- Ask for help and support from loved ones.

Medication Treatment of Bipolar Disorder

Medications used in bipolar disorder are intended to treat acute episodes of mania or depression, and also to prevent future episodes from occurring. These medications are referred to by various terms; mood stabilizers, antimanic agents or anticycling agents. In general, these are interchangeable terms.

Antidepressants are also used to treat bipolar disorder for depressive episodes, if a mood stabilizer alone is not sufficient. If there are psychotic symptoms present, medications called antipsychotics, or neuroleptics (see chapter 8) may also be necessary. If the person is extremely anxious or agitated, an antianxiety medicine may also be prescribed (see chapter 7).

Mood Stabilizers and How They Work

The three most widely used mood stabilizers are lithium, carbamazepine, and valproate. Carbamazepine and valproate are anticonvulsants. Two newer anticonvulsants, gabapentin and lamotrigine, are currently being evaluated for potential usefulness in treating bipolar disorder. All of these medications work differently from each other. This means that for some people it will be necessary to try different medicines until the best one can be determined. It can also mean that if one mood stabilizer does not work well, there is a good chance that another one will. The mood stabilizers may begin to take effect within the first week of treatment. However, full stabilization of mood and behaviors can take up to eight weeks.

Research on Effectiveness

Most people experience some symptom relief with mood stabilizers. In the United States, lithium is the medication that has been most widely used since the early 1970s. There are many more studies on its effectiveness than there are for the other mood stabilizers. In general, about 60–80 percent of all people on lithium experience a significant reduction in their symptoms.

Of the anticonvulsants, valproate and carbamazepine have been used for a much longer period and have been studied more intensively than gabapentin and lamotrigine, which have been available only for a short time. Valproate and carbamazepine are very effective medications, especially for rapid cycling bipolar disorder or other difficult to treat cases.

It is becoming more common to see combinations of mood stabilizers used. There is also increasing evidence that the effectiveness of a mood stabilizer, or a combination, may change over the course of the disease for a given person. A medication that previously worked well for someone may begin to lose effectiveness for reasons that are not clearly understood.

As with all medications, side effects, drug interactions, or effects of the particular drug on an existing medical condition must be considered. With the mood stabilizers it is these factors that often determine which medication will work best for a given individual. Because the mood stabilizers differ so much from each other, we will discuss each one individually.

Lithium

Lithium is a basic element found on the Periodic Chart of Elements, in the same chemical family as sodium and potassium. Lithium shares some, but not all, of the properties of the other elements in its family. Although widely found in nature, a physiological function for lithium has not been discovered.

The exact way in which lithium works is not completely understood. Current research suggests that it works inside the nerve cells in the brain to stabilize overactive systems that regulate mood. These overactive circuits can lead to either mania or depression, depending on which system is affected. It appears that lithium can interrupt several overactive pathways, which may explain its effectiveness in treating both mania and depression.

Medication Treatment:
What to Expect

When lithium is initiated, the starting dose will be in the range of 600–900 mg per day. The dose will be gradually increased

over the first seven to ten days. During, and immediately following, the acute manic phase, the dose will be kept at about
1200–2400 mg daily. After the acute episode has resolved, many
patients will not need as much lithium. The dose during the maintenance phase will be between 600–1800 mg per day. Lithium is
available as following products:

**Tablets or capsules, as lithium carbonate (not extended re-
lease)**

- Eskalith 300 mg tablets and 300 mg capsules
- Lithonate 300 mg capsules
- Lithotabs 300 mg tablets
- Various generic products available in 150 mg, 300 mg, and 600
  mg tablets or capsules

Extended release tablets, as lithium carbonate

- Eskalith CR 450 mg tablets
- Lithobid 300 mg tablets

Syrup, as lithium citrate

- Cibalith-S 300 mg/teaspoonful (sugar free)*
- Various generic products 300 mg/teaspoonful*

The best way to ensure that the dosage of lithium is correct
for someone is to measure the amount of lithium in the blood.
This is necessary because lithium can have some very serious side
effects, which are often related to its level in the bloodstream. The
amount of lithium required to produce symptom relief is very
close to the amount that can be dangerously high, or toxic. To
avoid problems with a high blood level of lithium, laboratory tests
are performed periodically to make sure the range is both safe and
effective. It is important to discuss the frequency of these laboratory tests with the doctor who is prescribing lithium. The dosages
and blood level values for lithium are summarized below:

	Dosage Range	Blood Level
Acute mania	1200–2400 mg/day	0.8–1.5 mEq/L
Maintenance	600–1800 mg/day	0.6–1.2 mEq/L

---

* Contains alcohol.

Side Effects

To get the most benefit from treatment with lithium it is extremely important to have an understanding of the side effects. Many side effects are not serious and can be effectively managed. Others can be more serious. All side effects should be reported to the doctor. If the side effects are severe, they should be reported immediately. The following information is not inclusive and is intended to give only a general idea of what to watch for.

- *Nausea, vomiting, diarrhea*—These can occur to varying degrees and at any time during treatment. These side effects can be minimized by taking lithium with food or meals. Sometimes the long-acting forms of lithium will produce fewer of these gastrointestinal symptoms. *However, if these symptoms are severe, or arise suddenly after someone has been taking lithium for some time, who has not previously been bothered by these side effects, the doctor should be notified immediately.*

- *Tremor of the hands*—Many people will experience a slight tremor in the hands when lithium is first started. This usually goes away with time. Limiting or avoiding caffeine helps lessen this tremor. Other medications can sometimes be added to help reduce a tremor. *If this hand tremor becomes more noticeable or appears suddenly, the doctor should be notified.*

- *Drowsiness, fatigue*—When people first start taking lithium they may experience some degree of drowsiness or sedation. Usually, this is not severe, although caution is advised when driving. For most people, this side effect disappears. *However, if a person is noticeably sedated, appears confused, has slurred speech or difficulty walking, the doctor should be notified immediately.* People often report feeling "slowed down" while taking lithium. This is a different sensation than the drowsiness described above. Sometimes this just means that the symptoms of mania or hypomania are responding to treatment. As mentioned earlier, some people do not like to lose the manic high and will use this effect as a reason to stop taking lithium.

- *Effects on kidneys*—Lithium relies on the kidney to be removed from the body. Keeping the kidneys functioning well by drinking lots of fluids helps to ensure that lithium is removed from the body properly. Lithium can cause increased urination and thirst, which go away for most people. *Anytime a person becomes dehydrated, or loses sodium from the body, there is a potential for lithium levels to increase. People can become dehydrated from having the flu, running a fever, sweating excessively, or taking certain medications. The doctor prescribing lithium should be informed of any of the above-mentioned situations.*

- *Effects on the thyroid gland*—Lithium can cause a change in some laboratory tests that are used to measure thyroid function. For most people, this is not significant. A small number of people experience a decrease in the functioning of the thyroid gland (hypothyroidism). The doctor may decide that supplementing the lithium with a thyroid medication is the best approach, or may try another mood stabilizer.

- *Weight gain*—Weight gain, from five to twenty pounds, may occur while taking lithium. This side effect will cause some people to want to stop the medication.

- *Rash or acne*—Either or both can result from taking lithium. If the rash and/or acne are severe enough, the lithium may need to be stopped.

Carbamazepine

Carbamazepine (brand-name Tegretol) has been used for more than twenty-five years to treat bipolar disorder. This medicine is chemically related to the tricyclic antidepressants. The exact way in which carbamazepine works has not been identified. It has been widely studied, without yielding conclusive results, to support the theory that it works by reducing the kindling process. As described previously, kindling is a process by which the brain becomes increasingly sensitized to various stimuli and, eventually, spontaneous abnormal brain activity occurs. Carbamazepine also affects the regulation of the movement of sodium and potassium in and out of nerve cells. And, like lithium, it can stabilize malfunctioning neurotransmitter circuits inside cells.

Medication Treatment:
What to Expect

When carbamazepine is initiated, the starting dose will be in the range of 200–400 mg per day. Over the first two to three weeks, the dose will be increased to a range of 600–1600 mg daily. Smaller, more gradual increases in dosage can help keep side effects to a minimum. The amount of carbamazepine in the bloodstream must be measured periodically. The level that is safe and effective for most people is 4–10 mcg/ml. This drug is available as the following products:

- Carbamazepine 100 mg chewable tablets (as common brand-name, Tegretol)

- Carbamazepine 200 mg tablets (as generic and common brand-name, Tegretol)

- Tegretol XR (extended release) 100 mg, 200 mg and 400 mg tablets

- Liquid, 100 mg/teaspoonful

Side Effects

- *Stomach upset*—Nausea, vomiting, diarrhea, and stomach cramps can occur. These side effects can be minimized by taking the dose with food or milk.

- *Sedation and drowsiness*—Most noticeable when the drug is first started; for most people, these side effects go away. *Dizziness* and *blurred vision* are also possible.

- *Skin*—A red, itching rash, or hives, may develop. Sometimes it does not go away and the drug must be stopped. Carbamazepine also can increase the skin's sensitivity to sunlight, leading to sunburn or discoloration. The use of sunscreen is recommended.

- *Heart rate*—The heart rate can become slowed with carbamazepine. This is most likely to be a problem for older people.

- *Effects on blood*—Although rare in adults, carbamazepine can cause anemia, or lower the red blood cell or white blood cell count.

- *Effects on the liver*—Carbamazepine can cause damage to the liver, but this is a rare occurrence. Laboratory tests can be done to monitor for this.

Valproate

Valproate, also called valproic acid, and known by the brand-names Depakote and Depakene, has been used for about twenty years in the treatment of bipolar disorder. The precise manner in which valproate works has not been determined. One of its strongest effects is on a neurotransmitter called GABA. It is thought that valproate increases the GABA levels in the brain, which leads to decreasing manic symptoms.

Medication Treatment: What to Expect

When valproate treatment is initiated, the starting dose will be in the range of 500–750 mg per day. Sometimes the starting dose can be higher as long as the person does not experience serious side effects, especially stomach upset. The dose will be increased over the first one to two weeks to 750–1500 mg daily. The amount of valproate in the bloodstream will be measured periodically. The level that is safe and effective for most people is 50–100 mcg/ml. This drug is available as the following products:

- Divalproex sodium, 125 mg, 250 mg, 500 mg delayed-release tablets (brand name Depakote)

- Divalproex sodium, 125 mg sprinkle capsules (brand-name Depakote)

- Valproic acid 250 mg capsules (generic and brand-name Depakene)

- Valproic acid, liquid, 250 mg/teaspoonful (generic and brand-name Depakene)

Side Effects

- *Stomach upset*—Nausea, vomiting, and indigestion are common, although usually not severe, and diminish with time. The delayed-release tablet form is less likely to cause stomach upset than are the capsules. Rarely, valproate can cause pain and inflammation in the pancreas. The sign that this may be occurring is severe abdominal pain. *Notify your physician immediately if you experience sudden, very intense abdominal pain.*

- *Dizziness, moderate drowsiness, hand tremor*—These side effects are usually not significant and will go away with time. *However, if a person is noticeably sedated, appears confused, has slurred speech or difficulty walking, the doctor should be notified immediately.*

- *Tremor of the hands*—Many people will experience a slight tremor in the hands when valproate is first started. This usually goes away with time. Limiting or avoiding caffeine will help to lessen this tremor. Other medications sometimes can be added to help reduce a tremor.

- *Weight gain or loss*—This is usually accompanied by an increase or decrease in appetite.

- *Hair loss*—This may be a short-term effect.

- *Effects on blood*—Although rare, sometimes the normal manner in which blood clots may be inhibited. The result can be increased bleeding and/or bruising.

- *Effects on the liver*—Rarely, valproate can cause damage to the liver. Laboratory tests should be done to monitor for this possibility.

New Anticonvulsants

A brief discussion of two new drugs, gabapentin and lamotrigine, follows. Time will tell whether either or both of these will play an important part in the treatment of bipolar disorder.

Gabapentin

This medication, marketed under the brand name of Neurontin, is thought to have an effect on the GABA neurotransmitter system. It is not clear whether this action explains how it might be helpful in bipolar disorder. The dose of gabapentin is usually 300–400 mg per day. Blood level monitoring is not necessary for this drug. Common side effects are drowsiness, tremor, and blurred vision.

Lamotrigine

This medication, with the brand-name of Lamictal, is assumed to work by decreasing the effects of an excitatory neurotransmitter called glutamate. This may or may not explain how it works in treating bipolar disorder. The dose of lamotrigine is 200–500 mg daily. Blood level monitoring is recommended. The common side effects are drowsiness, headache, blurred vision, stomach upset, and skin rash.

Precautions and Contraindications

Some general precautions apply to the mood stabilizers. None is considered absolutely safe during pregnancy. All carry particular risks to the fetus, and their use should be avoided if possible, particularly in the first three months of gestation. However, if a pregnant woman's bipolar illness is extremely serious, and there are no other alternatives, it may be necessary for her to take a mood stabilizer. This should be done only under very close management by a doctor.

Lithium is generally not recommended for people who have kidney disease. The anticonvulsants should be used cautiously if there is liver damage or kidney disease.

Caution: There can be serious consequences if these medications are taken in very high doses, as in accidental or intentional overdoses. An overdose of lithium is especially dangerous and can be fatal if levels are extremely high. There is no known antidote for a serious lithium overdose. There are severe consequences to overdose of all the anticonvulsant medicines, as well. Serious overdoses can lead to death.

Because antidepressants frequently are prescribed for the depressed phase of bipolar disorder, it is important to be aware that antidepressants can be associated with triggering manic or hypomanic episodes, sometimes called a "manic switch." Such occurrences are infrequent. It is generally believed that the tricyclics are the most likely group to have this effect, although it is also possible with the SSRIs. Among antidepressants, Bupropion and the MAO-inhibitors are considered to pose less of a risk for a "manic switch" to occur.

There are important drug-drug interactions to be aware of with the mood stabilizers. These are outlined in Part II of this book. If you are seeing more than one doctor, make sure each is physician is aware of all the medications you are taking. Checking with a doctor or pharmacist before using any over-the-counter medication is strongly advised.

Alcohol should be avoided while taking any mood stabilizer. Even moderate use is not recommended, and chronic use is potentially dangerous. Additional sedative effects can occur when the mood stabilizers are combined with alcohol. Also, because alcohol can cause mood changes, the effectiveness of the mood stabilizers may be decreased. Potentially, alcoholism can damage the liver, which also means that the body will have more difficulty metabolizing the anticonvulsant mood stabilizers.

Are Mood Stabilizers Addictive or Habit-Forming?

None of the mood stabilizers are known to cause tolerance, dependence, or addiction. However, some of the antianxiety medications (e.g., Valium) that are used in conjunction with the mood stabilizers do have the potential to cause addiction. These medicines should be used with caution if the patient has a history of alcohol or drug abuse.

Another area for concern arises when someone in a manic episode uses prescribed medications inappropriately in an attempt to maintain the "high" of mania. Even if these medicines do not have the properties of abusable substances, the poor judgment characteristic of a manic episode can lead a person to take doses or combinations of medications in ways not intended, under the mistaken assumption that the high can be achieved. Sometimes the result can be that a person ingests dangerously high doses or unsafe combinations of a variety of medications.

What if the First-Line Treatment Is Not Successful?

For most people, the mood stabilizers will begin to work within the first week. Over the next six to seven weeks there should be noticeable and progressive improvement in symptoms. If this expected progression does not happen, there are several steps to follow:

- Verify the diagnosis of bipolar disorder
- Determine that the medication regimen is being followed
- Identify current medications that might be causing persisting symptoms
- Rule out any substance or alcohol abuse

Once these issues have been satisfactorily addressed, if the dose of any of the medications can be safely increased, such an increase, with careful monitoring, may be prescribed. Because increasing the dose can lead to more side effects, another strategy, called *augmentation*, may be used.

Usually, with augmentation, a second mood stabilizer is added. An antidepressant also can be added if the persisting symptoms are depressive in nature. If there are persistent manic or hypomanic symptoms, an evaluation of the current medications may reveal that it is prudent to stop one of the medications. This can be a very frustrating time for those who have a hard time controlling symptoms in spite of many medication changes. It is important to evaluate where in the lifetime course of the disorder the person is located. There is some evidence that, as the course of bipolar disorder worsens over time, medications may lose effectiveness.

Electroconvulsive Therapy

If repeated medication trials fail, or are contraindicated, electroconvulsive therapy (ECT) is an alternative treatment. For both manic and depressed phases, ECT can be extremely effective and provide prompt results. The modern methods by which ECT is administered are very safe.

Other Treatments for Bipolar Disorder

Following are brief accounts of other treatments that are sometimes used or discussed for bipolar disorder. The results from most of these treatments have not been widely studied, and they may or may not hold strong hope as potential treatments. We think it is important to mention them in case you see other references to them. They are almost always reserved for very difficult cases of bipolar disorder. It is important to reiterate that these therapies do not have an established place among standard treatments. However, if your doctor is considering one of these therapies, it may be a reasonable choice if other alternatives have failed.

Calcium Channel Blockers

Usually, these medications are used to treat cardiac conditions and high blood pressure. There has been some interest in their role in treating bipolar disorder. The two medicines most often discussed are verapamil and nimodipine.

Atypical Antipsychotics

See chapter 8 for a full discussion of these agents. The two that have received some attention are clozapine and risperidone.

Anxiety Disorders

Introduction

Anxiety is a part of life. Indeed, it is hard-wired into our brains. When people feel anxious or threatened, they are likely to respond with an increase in tension and the physiological arousal that has been called the "fight-or-flight response." This is an automatic biological response that prepares us for action. The basic paradigm of the fight-or-flight response is that of prehistoric hunters confronted by a saber-toothed tiger. They must act quickly either by attacking the tiger or fleeing, both actions requiring rapid mobilization of energy and alertness. This is a life-saving response; that is why it evolved and continues to exist some 30,000 years after the extinction of saber-toothed tigers.

In modern life, however, this fight-or-flight response can go awry. For example, people with anxiety disorders can experience the full set of these biological reactions without an actual threat being present. That is, their hearts beat faster, their lungs breathe more oxygen, they sweat more, their pupils dilate, their hands and feet tingle and go numb from decreased blood flow, and they produce and secrete adrenaline and other stress hormones in larger amounts.

In today's world we are rarely faced with real physical danger. But we are biologically programmed to react to *stress* itself.

This means that our bodies react to the many stresses of modern life as if they were physical threats, like tigers, instead of financial woes or deadline pressures. In addition, many people have an exaggerated physiological and psychological response even to minor stresses. People suffering from some anxiety disorders often experience the complete physiological fight-or-flight response even in the absence of any stressful event.

Anxiety Disorders

There are several types of anxiety disorders, including situational anxiety, phobias, social phobia, panic disorder, generalized anxiety disorder, and obsessive-compulsive disorder. The distinctions between these various types of anxiety depend on whether the anxiety is brief or constant, and whether it is generalized (i.e., experienced in all situations) or specific to a particular situation. *Situational anxiety* refers to what is often simply called "stress." It is an overly anxious reaction to a situation. *Phobias* refer to an exaggerated fear of a particular thing, such as a phobia of spiders, or a fear of flying in an airplane. *Social phobia* refers to intense anxiety about social situations. *Panic disorder* is distinguished by the sufferer experiencing sudden attacks of very severe anxiety that last for only a few minutes. *Generalized anxiety disorder* manifests as a near-constant anxiety. And, *obsessive-compulsive disorder* is distinguished by compulsive, ritualistic behaviors and/or frightening thoughts (e.g., fears regarding dirt, germs, and contamination).

Altogether these disorders affect between 10 and 20 percent of the population at any given time, and some 20–25 percent of people over their lifespans (Kessler et al. 1994). In their more severe forms, anxiety disorders cause tremendous suffering, are very disabling, and are sometimes associated with suicide. Often some of the symptoms begin in childhood, so that the person has a life-long struggle with anxiety. In this chapter we will take a separate look at each type of anxiety disorder, and its medical treatment.

Medical Causes of Anxiety

Sometimes anxiety can be caused by a physical reason. These can include various medical conditions and certain drugs. Hyperthyroidism is one of the more common physical causes of anxiety. When the thyroid gland is overactive, it can produce symptoms that mimic an anxiety disorder, such as tremulousness, feelings of anxiety, and rapid heart rate. The following medical disorders have been associated with anxiety.

Disorders that May Cause Anxiety

- Adrenal tumor
- Alcoholism

- Angina pectoris
- Cardiac arrhythmia
- CNS degenerative disease
- Cushing's disease
- Coronary insufficiency
- Delirium*

- Hyperthyroidism
- Ménière's disease (early stages)
- Parathyroid disease
- Partial-complex seizures
- Postconcussion syndrome
- Premenstrual syndrome
- Pulmonary embolism
- Mitral valve prolapse**

In addition, many drugs can cause anxiety. Among them are amphetamines, asthma medications, caffeine, central nervous system depressants, such as alcohol (withdrawal from), cocaine, nasal decongestants, steroids, and appetite suppressants.

In the initial evaluation of an anxiety disorder, it is always a good idea to have a physical examination, including appropriate laboratory tests, and to give a thorough drug history, including prescription, over-the-counter, and street drugs. If a medical condition or drug usage is found, it is important to first treat the underlying disorder that may be causing the anxiety or to address the drug use. Then, if necessary, treatment targeted specifically at anxiety can begin.

---

* Delirium can occur as a result of many toxic and metabolic conditions and often produces anxiety and agitation.

** The mitral valve prolapse (MVP) does not cause anxiety, but it has been found that MVP and anxiety disorders often coexist. This may be due to some common underlying genetic factor.

Situational Anxiety—Adjustment Disorder with Anxiety

Diagnosis: To understand this type of anxiety disorder better, we need to examine the fight-or-flight response more closely. As stated earlier, our brains are hard-wired to react to stress in a particular way.

A stressful event evokes both a thinking response in the cortex, and an emotional response in the limbic system. The limbic system then, with input from the cortex, induces a multitude of physiological changes, as described above, including a release of stress hormones, which prepares us for action. *People experience these physiological changes as anxiety.*

At mild or moderate levels, situational anxiety is usually well tolerated and prepares us to perform better. However, when an event is particularly stressful, we may experience severe or overwhelming anxiety. The same event may be more stressful to some people than to others, usually due to one's previous experiences, which color the way in which the event is viewed. Also, some people may become alarmed by their reaction and thereby compound their anxiety.

For example, when interviewing for a job, most people tend to be somewhat anxious. If, however, they react to this anxiety with alarm, thinking they are sure to do poorly in the interview, this will increase their anxiety and they will be more likely to appear anxious and to stumble over their words. This type of situational anxiety is usually self-limiting and eventually dissipates as the stressful event recedes into the past.

Medical Treatment

The usual medical treatment for situational anxiety is antianxiety medication, also called "minor tranquilizers." These medications have been used since the mid-1950s to treat anxiety. They are usually very effective at relieving it and have few side effects. The main side effects they do have are sedation and a tendency to increase the effects of other drugs, such as alcohol. They also can be habit-forming if used for more than a few weeks. Some of these medications have achieved notoriety because of this side effect, as described in the book *I'm Dancing as Fast as I Can* (Gordon 1990). The following chart shows a list of the drugs in this class.

Dosages of Antianxiety Agents

Generic Name	Brand-Name	Single-Dose Dosage Range (mg)	Usual Dosage Range (mg/day)
Minor Tranquilizers			
Diazepam	Valium	2–10	4–40
Chlordiazepoxide	Librium	10–50	15–100
Flurazepam	Dalmane	15–60	15–60
Prazepam	Centrax	5–30	20–40
Clorazepate	Tranxene	3.75–15	7.5–60
Clonazepam	Klonopin	0.5–2	1–8
Temazepam	Restoril	15–30	15–60
Lorazepam	Ativan	0.5–2	1.5–6
Alprazolam	Xanax	0.25–2	0.5–6
Oxazepam	Serax	10–30	30–90
Triazolam	Halcion	0.125–0.5	0.125–0.5
Midazolam	Versed (injectable only)	1–2.5	1–15
Quazepam	Doral	7.5–30	7.5–30
Other Antianxiety Medications			
Estazolam	ProSom	1.0–2.0	1.0–2.0
Zolpidem	Ambien	5–10	5–10
Buspirone	BuSpar	5–20	10–40
Hydroxyzine	Atarax, Vistaril	10–50	30–200
Diphenhydramine	Benadryl	25–100	75–200
Propranolol	Inderal	10–80	20–160
Atenolol	Tenormin	25–100	25–100
Clonidine	Catapres	0.1–0.3	0.2–0.9

Often, someone will be prescribed a minor tranquilizer to be taken when the anxiety is particularly severe. Thus, several doses may be taken on some days and none on others. Usually, these antianxiety medications can be used safely for two to five months without significant dependency developing, depending upon the individual. However, when used for more than six months, dependency is likely to develop. Over time, as the anxiety gradually diminishes, the medication can be used less frequently, and eventually discontinued.

Minor Tranquilizers

Minor tranquilizers are the most commonly prescribed antianxiety medications. In fact, at times, they have been the most commonly prescribed of all prescription medications. Their widespread use is due to their safety and effectiveness and to the ubiquity of anxiety disorders. These medications are very effective, approaching 100-percent effectiveness.

They work by binding to certain receptor sites in the brain associated with the neurotransmitter GABA. When they bind to this receptor they seem to reduce the reactiveness of the limbic system.

Caution: If these medications have been taken daily for several weeks or more, they should never be stopped abruptly because of the risk of serious withdrawal symptoms.

Treatment Considerations: What to Expect

In cases of situational anxiety, initially a low dose of medication may be prescribed. Typically, 0.5 to 1 mg of lorazepam, or the equivalent, is an effective starting dose, taken up to two to three times daily. For situational anxiety, however, it is usually not necessary to take the medication routinely. It can be taken when anxiety increases, or when an increase is anticipated. Sometimes, after a few weeks of use, the medication doesn't seem to work quite as well, and a small dosage increase may be necessary. This reduction in anxiety helps people to function better and thus allows time for them to address the situation that caused it. Then, over time, use of the medication can be gradually tapered off. The average length of treatment is a few weeks to a few months. In situational anxiety, insomnia, especially a difficulty in falling asleep, is often a problem. These medications have proved useful for dealing with this problem (on a short-term basis).

Side Effects

As a rule, if taken in the correct dose, minor tranquilizers are relatively free of side effects. However, the correct dose varies from person to person. It the dose is too low, the anxiety will still be noticeable. If the dose is too high, the person may feel drowsy or even drunk, talk with slurred speech, and walk unsteadily. Obviously, driving a car or operating machinery should not be attempted under these circumstances. If the dose is correct, however, people are usually able to drive, and do all of their customary activities. As with all medications, other reactions are possible. Some people may develop a rash. On very rare occasions some people react "paradoxically" and become more agitated instead of calmer.

Addiction Potential

Minor tranquilizers have an addiction potential similar to that of alcohol. When taken, they can create feelings that are like those experienced when drinking alcohol. They also have a withdrawal syndrome similar to alcohol. (Contrary to popular belief, alcohol can be habit-forming, but not everyone becomes dependent on it.) Most people can use minor tranquilizers in a controlled fashion, but some tend to become hooked on them. Fortunately, minor tranquilizers are not toxic to the brain, liver, and other organs as alcohol is. In general, they are very helpful for reducing suffering and they are safe, but must be used with caution.

Other Treatments

Minor tranquilizers are the mainstay of the treatment of situational anxiety, but other medications can be considered. These include the antihistamines and beta-blockers. The main antihistamine used for anxiety is hydroxyzine (Vistaril or Atarax). It is sedating and has some antianxiety effect. It is not habit-forming. The main problem with it is that often, in order to take enough to reduce anxiety, significant drowsiness may be produced. The usual starting dose is 10–25 mg three to four times daily. Beta-blockers are blood pressure medications that block the effects of adrenaline. They are better at reducing the physical symptoms of anxiety than the emotional feeling of anxiety. They can cause low blood pressure and light-headedness. The usual starting dose is 20–40 mg of propranolol, or the equivalent. They are not habit-forming, but should not be stopped abruptly because of the possibility of temporarily raising the person's blood pressure.

Psychological Treatments

Psychotherapy is often very helpful for treating situational anxiety. Discussing the stressful situation helps to reduce the anxiety response and different anxiety management strategies can be used to reduce the severity of the anxiety symptoms. Problem-solving discussions and learning how to use effective coping techniques can guide the anxiety sufferer to correct or alter stress-producing situations.

Are Medications Habit-Forming?

Drug Dependence: When some medications are taken on a regular basis, they may cause dependence. However, dependence is not the same as addiction. Dependence simply means that the body adapts to the medication, that is, the body gets used to the medication. When this occurs, if the medication is abruptly discontinued, there may be withdrawal symptoms (the body's reaction to a sudden chemical change). Depending on the medication, withdrawal symptoms can be fairly mild (e.g., a slight headache or nausea) or very severe (e.g., seizures).* Technically, drug dependence does not mean abuse or addiction.

Drug Addiction: Some medications have the potential for addiction (especially if the patient has a history of prior substance abuse). With addiction there is dependence (and withdrawal symptoms upon sudden discontinuation) and three important additional features:

- There may be drug-craving, i.e., a strong desire to use the drug to experience pleasure/euphoria.

---

* If medications that have a potential for dependence are discontinued very gradually, withdrawal symptoms can be avoided.

- There is a need to use higher and higher doses to achieve euphoria.
- The drug abuse continues even when it is apparent that it is causing health problems, occupational or academic failure, or serious interpersonal difficulties.

Medication Class	Dependence	Addiction Potential
Antidepressants	No[1]	No
Antianxiety medications	Yes	Yes[2]
Lithium	No	No
Antipsychotics	No	No
Stimulants	Yes	Yes[2]

Phobias

Diagnosis: *Phobias* are characterized by a fear of a particular object or situation. When someone who has a phobia is faced with the feared object or situation, this leads to increased anxiety and frequently to avoidance of the feared object or situation. Often this causes only minimal disruption, but it can be significant when a person's job requires exposure to the object of the phobia. For example, someone who has a phobia of flying in airplanes, but whose job involves a lot of travel, will be severely impacted by such a phobia.

Medical Treatment

Antianxiety medication can be used to reduce the anxiety experienced when the phobic person is exposed to the object of the phobia, thereby making the anxiety easier to tolerate. For example, someone with a fear of flying can take a minor tranquilizer just prior to boarding the plane (i.e., one hour before the flight). Once in flight, the anxiety usually diminishes, and the rest of the flight can be completed without excessive anxiety.

---

1 Antidepressants *may* have *mild* withdrawal symptoms. That is why almost always discontinuation is done gradually.
2 Generally, these medications are addictive only for those who have a personal or family history of alcohol or substance abuse.

Beta-blockers are another class of medication used to treat phobias. They can be used, for example, to treat a phobia of public speaking. As a rule, propranolol (10–20 mg) or atenolol (25–50 mg) taken thirty minutes before speaking will significantly reduce the jitters associated with public speaking. Beta-blockers have the effect of lowering blood pressure, but are not habit-forming, and in these low doses they usually do not have side effects.

Psychological Treatment

Psychological treatment is very important in the treatment of simple phobias. This usually involves a type of treatment referred to as *systematic desensitization*, in which the phobic person is repeatedly exposed to the phobic stimulus and gradually becomes more and more comfortable with it. Basically, it is impossible to truly overcome a phobia without facing the fear. The key is to do it gradually so that the anxiety is not severe, and to experience success in facing the feared situation a little at a time.

Social Phobia

Diagnosis: *Social phobia* refers to an exaggerated fear of social situations. People with social phobia are very anxious about being in social situations and will often avoid them as much as possible. When in a social situation, they experience severe anxiety and are plagued with thoughts about how the other people present are probably judging them in very negative ways. They often fear embarrassment or humiliation. Sometimes, people with social phobia may have occasional panic attacks in reaction to social situations. It is not uncommon for people with social phobia to use alcohol or antianxiety medications to control their anxiety. Studies suggest that between 5 and 10 percent of all people will experience social phobia at some time during their life (Kessler et al. 1994). This disorder causes significant degrees of distress and, at times, it leads to social isolation, depression, alcoholism, or drug abuse.

Medical Treatments

Two types of medication have shown promise in the treatment of social phobia: antidepressant and antianxiety drugs. The

MAO-inhibitor antidepressants are the most effective treatment. These medications, however, have significant serious side effects and therefore are not usually the first-line choice. Some recent studies have shown benefit from the SSRI antidepressants (Lydiard et al. 1995). These medications are safer than MAO-inhibitors and are usually well tolerated. MAO-inhibitors and SSRIs are discussed in greater detail in chapter 5. Antianxiety medications frequently are helpful, but they must be used with caution because social phobia is usually a chronic condition and continual use of these medications leads to dependency and at times leads to abuse.

Psychological Treatments

The most effective treatment for social phobia is group psychotherapy. In a group, the phobic person is faced with his/her specific social anxiety and has the opportunity within the group structure to develop more effective social skills. The group provides a chance to practice interacting in a supportive setting. However, this often necessitates long-term group treatment.

Panic Disorder

Diagnosis: *Panic disorder* is characterized by acute attacks of anxiety, which are so severe that sufferers often fear they will go crazy or die. These attacks come on very suddenly, are very intense, and last from a few minutes to an hour. The attacks are accompanied by any number of the following physical symptoms:

- Shortness of breath
- Fear of losing control or going crazy
- Tingling (usually of the hands)
- Feeling of choking
- Chills or hot flushes
- Sweating
- Fear of dying

- Tremulousness or restlessness
- Rapid heartbeat or palpitations
- Light-headedness and dizziness
- Nausea or abdominal distress
- Chest pain or discomfort
- Feeling of unreality

Typically, panic disorder will begin with a single, isolated panic attack. (See Jill's Case in chapter 1.) This attack is so frightening that the person often becomes anxious and fearful about having another attack. He or she develops significant anticipatory anxiety about having another attack and may begin, therefore, to experience anxiety most of the time.

Such people often come to feel more secure at home and develop phobias about traveling any distance away from home. They are uncomfortable especially when they feel trapped and are unable to go home immediately, as in heavy traffic or in a crowd. Thus, people with panic disorder go from having discrete anxiety attacks, to having near-constant anxiety and phobias of specific activities, punctuated by periodic full-blown panic attacks. This can progress to *agoraphobia*, a condition where the fears are so pervasive and intense that the person essentially becomes housebound.

Panic Disorder and the Brain

Panic disorder is probably caused by a dysregulation of the neurochemical, norepinephrine, such that a large amount of norepinephrine is released very suddenly. Norepinephrine is an adrenaline-like compound that is released in the brain and body during the flight-or-fight response. It produces increased heart rate, elevated blood pressure, and other physical symptoms of anxiety. Evidence suggests that in panic disorder, there is an abnormality in the part of the brain called the locus coeruleus (Redmond 1985). The locus coeruleus (LC) stimulates the release of norepinephrine in other parts of the brain. It appears that, in those who have panic disorder, the LC overreacts to even minor stimuli. It is as if their LC has a hair trigger so delicate that a small stimulus produces a strong reaction. In addition, people with panic disorder tend to have higher than normal resting levels of anxiety/norepinephrine so that they tend to be always on the verge of a panic attack.

Medical Treatment

Panic disorder is usually treated with minor tranquilizers and/or antidepressants. Minor tranquilizers, or antianxiety medications, offer the advantage of working quickly and having few side effects. Unfortunately, they have the problem of being habit-forming. Antidepressants, on the other hand, are slow to work, and often have multiple side effects but they are not habit--forming. Other medications, such beta-blockers and buspirone, may be helpful as adjuncts to the treatment, but they are not first-line treatments.

Initially, minor tranquilizers often are used to gain quick control over the panic attacks, which are frequently intolerable and debilitating. Then, an antidepressant may be added. The antidepressant must be started at a very low dose, because this often increases anxiety at the start. The starting dose may be as low as 5 mg or less of fluoxetine, or 10 mg of imipramine. (See table 5.1 "Antidepressants at a Glance" in chapter 5.) They may take up to six weeks to begin to have significant benefit. Then the dose of the minor tranquilizer can be reduced gradually and, hopefully, soon discontinued. As a rule, medication must be continued for one to three years, but some people must take it indefinitely because they experience a return of symptoms whenever the dosage is reduced.

Psychological Treatment

Psychotherapy, particularly *cognitive-behavioral* therapy, can be very helpful in treating panic disorder. Treatment for panic disorder can be seen as having two phases: first, medication and/or cognitive-behavioral treatment for the panic attacks per se, and then cognitive-behavioral treatment for the associated phobias. Once the frequency and severity of the panic attacks have been reduced, gradually panic disorder sufferers will experience less anticipatory anxiety about having a panic attack.

They can then begin to confront some of their phobias, secure in the knowledge that they are not likely to have a panic attack. Often, however, panic attacks cannot be entirely eliminated, and it is important that people become able to talk themselves through a panic attack, to reduce their anxiety levels while they wait for the panic attack to gradually subside. Cognitive therapy and/or relaxation training is often helpful for this.

Although strenuous exercise infrequently precipitates a panic attack, in the long run it is extremely helpful in reducing the frequency of the attacks. It is also important to avoid drugs that have stimulant properties, as they may induce panic attacks. These drugs include caffeine and decongestants such as phenylpropanolamine and pseudoephedrine.

Generalized Anxiety Disorder

Diagnosis: Generalized Anxiety Disorder (GAD) is characterized by almost constant anxiety. People suffering from this disorder are nervous most of the time regardless of the situation. They tend to be preoccupied about things that might go wrong. This makes any situation that is the least challenging much more difficult because of the associated anxiety and worry. This anxiety is accompanied by the following symptoms:

• Restlessness or feeling keyed up or on edge • Easily fatigued • Difficulty concentrating or mind going blank • Irritability • Muscle tension • Sleep disturbance, especially difficulty in falling asleep

Generalized Anxiety Disorder and the Brain

The etiology of Generalized Anxiety Disorder is not well understood at this time. One significant observation is that many people with GAD go on to develop clinical depression. It is likely that there is some imbalance involving the serotonin and/or norepinephrine systems. It is as though, physiologically, these people are in a perpetual state of the fight-or-flight response.

Medical Treatment

Psychological factors are often important in GAD and psychotherapy is often helpful for reducing symptoms. Three types of medication are most frequently used in the treatment of GAD: minor tranquilizers, buspirone, and antidepressants. As noted earlier, minor tranquilizers are antianxiety medications that reduce anxiety within thirty minutes of ingestion. They are habit-forming, so that their use in a chronic disorder is controversial. However, some people are able to take a stable dose daily for many years with significant benefit and no apparent adverse effects (Hollister 1993). Other people tend to use higher and higher doses and are prone to abusing these medications. Clearly, in such cases, the use of minor tranquilizers is not indicated. Those who are particularly prone to abuse are usually people with a history of alcohol or drug abuse, or those with blood relatives who have a history of alcohol or drug abuse.

Buspirone is a first-line medication treatment used particularly for GAD. It is an antianxiety medication, but one that is quite different from the minor tranquilizers. Buspirone is not habit-forming, but requires one to two weeks (or longer) before results are seen. The most common side effects are nausea, dizziness, headache and, paradoxically, occasionally, anxiety. These side effects tend to subside after two to three weeks. The usual starting dose for buspirone is 5 to 10 mg twice daily. Antidepressants, except for bupropion, may also be helpful in GAD. Beta-blockers and hydroxyzine, too, are helpful for some.

Psychological Treatment

Various types of therapy are often useful in treating GAD. These include the more traditional "talk therapy" and cognitive-behavioral therapy. Treatment is often a slow process, it may last many months.

Obsessive-Compulsive Disorder

Diagnosis: Obsessive-Compulsive Disorder (OCD) is characterized by obsessional thoughts and/or compulsive behaviors. Obsessional thoughts are intrusive thoughts that are very distressing to the person thinking them. They evoke a great deal of fearful anxiety, e.g., fears about oneself or loved ones becoming ill, infected with deadly viruses, or dying.

Compulsive behaviors are ritualistic behaviors that the person feels compelled to perform to ward off some impending calamity, or to reduce the feeling of intense anxiety. Examples include, checking locks, compulsive counting, tapping a certain number of times, positioning objects in specific ways, or excessive hand washing.

When the disorder is severe, much of the OCD person's time is occupied by the symptoms, so that performing even a simple task can become very time-consuming.

Obsessive-Compulsive Disorder and the Brain

Obsessive-Compulsive Disorder appears to be caused by a serotonin imbalance. PET scans show increased metabolic activity in the prefrontal cortex in the brain. Interestingly, these abnormalities tend to normalize during treatment, whether treatment is cognitive-behavioral therapy, pharmacological, or a combination of both.

Medical Treatment

Serotonin antidepressants are the most effective treatment used for OCD. These include the SSRIs and clomipramine. (See table 5.1 in chapter 5.) Other medications, such as minor tranquilizers and buspirone, may be helpful as adjuncts to first-line treatments. Treatment for anxiety with these antidepressants is similar to the treatment of depression. However, higher doses often may be required to control the symptoms, e.g., 60 to 80 mg per day of fluoxetine, or the equivalent.

Psychological Treatment

Cognitive-behavioral therapy is also very effective and may be combined with medication. The most effective treatment for reducing compulsive behaviors appears to be cognitive-behavioral therapy.

Psychotic Disorders

Introduction

Psychotic disorders are considered to be among the most serious mental illnesses. The term "psychosis" refers to a condition in which there is a significant loss of touch with consensual reality, and the creation of a new personal reality. Thus, people who are psychotic not only have lost touch with what is actually happening, but they often develop very surreal or bizarre thoughts about what is occurring, e.g., "Aliens have installed hidden cameras in my home."

There are a number of different forms of psychosis, or psychotic disorders. These include schizophrenia, psychotic depression, manic psychosis, atypical psychosis, and the organic psychoses. (When the psychosis is caused by a medical condition, such as Alzheimer's disease or a stroke, it is called an organic psychosis.) Many medical conditions can cause psychotic symptoms, for example, brain tumors, dementia, and hormone problems can cause psychosis, but a discussion of these specific illnesses is beyond the scope of this book. The focus in this chapter is on schizophrenia and similar psychoses.

Schizophrenia is considered a prototypical psychotic disorder. The name does *not* mean split personality or multiple personality disorder, as is sometimes thought. *Schizophrenia* means "split mind" and refers to a disorder characterized by hallucinations, delusions, and disorganized thinking. It affects approximately one percent of the population (APA 1994a). Schizophrenia is found in all countries and all cultures, and has been recognized since the time of Hippocrates. It often, but not always, leads to a chronic, disabling condition. New medication treatments, however, offer renewed hope for the treatment of this condition.

Diagnosis

The diagnosis of schizophrenia is made more on the basis of the course of the illness than on the person's condition at any one point in time. The course includes the initial (*prodromal*) phase when the person tends to become more withdrawn and has difficulties concentrating and performing daily activities. Often, during this phase, it may be misdiagnosed as depression. If this happens, the next phase, the *acute* phase, reveals the true nature of the illness.

In the acute phase, the person becomes floridly psychotic, behaving in a markedly different manner from his or her usual way of functioning; a way that is usually judged by others as bizarre or crazy. He or she may talk in a very irrational manner and say things that are clearly unbelievable. Later, usually after some type of treatment, people with schizophrenia enter what is called the *residual* phase, where symptoms are less severe. As in the prodromal phase, in the residual phase, sufferers may seem quiet, subdued, or depressed.

Making the Diagnosis

Some of the important markers of schizophrenia are as follow:

- The course of the illness, including the prodromal, active, and residual phases, must last longer than six months. In cases where the person recovers in less than six months, the diagnosis is *schizophreniform disorder*.

- During the acute phase, certain key symptoms must be present for a diagnosis of schizophrenia to be made correctly. The acute phase is the phase that must be distinguished from other types of psychosis. Manic psychosis and psychotic depression may appear to be similar to schizophrenia. The key differences between each illness are seen in the differences in mood changes.

- *Manic psychosis* is accompanied by a strong elevation of mood, such as euphoria, or anger, but it may be indistinguishable from the acute phase of schizophrenia.

- *Psychotic depression* includes the full array of clinical depression symptoms, which precede the development of psychotic depression symptoms. In this disorder, a person first becomes depressed and then develops psychotic symptoms. These symptoms often involve guilt and/or medical concerns. For example, some people believe that they hear voices, which tell them they deserve to die because they are so bad and worthless. Others might believe that they have developed undetected brain tumors or stomach cancers.

- *Atypical psychosis* and *delusional disorder* are less severe than the disorders discussed above, involving little disorganization of thinking. Furthermore, they usually do not last as long. Certain drugs (stimulants and hallucinogens) and some medical diseases can cause syndromes that mimic schizophrenia.

Signs and Symptoms

The signs and symptoms of schizophrenia are grouped into four types: positive, negative, disorganization, and characterological.

Positive symptoms include hallucinations, delusions, agitation, floridly bizarre behavior, and "first-rank" symptoms, which can include the belief that one is broadcasting one's thoughts to the world and/or the belief that one's thoughts, feelings, and actions are being controlled by an external agent.

Negative symptoms include anhedonia (the inability to feel pleasure), apathy, blunted affect, poverty of thought, feelings of emptiness, and a complete lack of imagination.

Disorganization symptoms include behavioral disorganization, distractibility, and thought disorder (i.e, marked confusion).

"Characterological" symptoms include social isolation or alienation, marked feelings of inadequacy, and poorly developed social skills.

Hallucinations and Delusions

When a person hears, sees, or smells something that *is not there*, as in hearing voices or seeing visions, that is called an *hallucination*. *Delusions* are false beliefs, a belief in something that is not true. These delusions might be something that *could be true*, such as, "I am being followed by the FBI." But, in schizophrenia, they are often quite bizarre, such as, "Martians have installed electro-magnetic lasers in my apartment and are broadcasting informa-tion about Earth to their leaders."

Because schizophrenia so profoundly alters a person's think-ing, the person often has a distorted view of what is happening to him or her. Friends and family are often more aware of these pro-found changes than the person with schizophrenia and they may see the need for treatment much more clearly than the person does. Someone with schizophrenia may deny that he or she is ill or tend to minimize the problem. When this occurs, that person may be quite resistant to treatment, thus making the process of obtaining treatment difficult. This can be especially hard on family members, as they try to encourage the person to cooperate with treatment.

Other Considerations

Schizophrenia must be distinguished from a psychosis caused by a medical illness or drugs. Where drug use is suspected, a urine drug screen can be helpful. Usually, medical illnesses have other symptoms that will show up in a physical examination or laboratory test. A century ago, neurosyphilis was a common cause of psychosis. Today, it has all but disappeared; nevertheless, it should be checked for by an easy laboratory test. And, as stated above, brain tumors, dementing illnesses, and hormone problems can also cause psychosis. The causes of organic psychoses are le-gion, but they can be grouped into the following types:

Causes of Organic Psychoses

- Metabolic
- Organ failure, such as kidney failure
- Hypoxia (oxygen deficiency)
- Hypoglycemia (insufficient blood sugar)
- Vitamin deficiency
- Endocrinopathy, such as hyperthyroidism
- Fluid or electrolyte imbalance
- Porphyria (abnormalities of porphyrin metabolism)
- Drug or alcohol intoxication or withdrawal
- Infections

- Epilepsy

- Head injury

- Vascular diseases, such as lupus

- Intracranial tumor

- Cerebral degenerative diseases
  Dementias, such as Alzheimer's disease
  Multiple sclerosis
  Huntington's chorea
  Parkinson's disease

Schizophrenia and the Brain

In recent years, an accumulating body of evidence has demonstrated important differences between the normal brain and the brains of people with schizophrenia. In the schizophrenic brain several types of changes have been noted such as, particular parts of the brain associated with information processing have been shown to be underdeveloped. Decreased metabolic activity in the prefrontal cortex, which correlates with the severity of negative symptoms, has been demonstrated. And increased dopamine (a neurochemical) activity, which correlates with the severity of positive symptoms, has been shown. How these changes produce the symptoms of schizophrenia is a matter of much theorizing at this point.

Antipsychotic Medications: What They Are and How They Work

Antipsychotic medications help to reduce psychotic symptoms. They are often used in schizophrenia, but they will treat psychotic symptoms regardless of the cause of the psychosis. They are somewhat sedating, but this is not how they work. Antipsychotic medications specifically target psychotic symptoms, especially delusions, hallucinations, and disorganized thinking. Until recently, they all worked by blocking dopamine in certain parts of the brain. Now, there are newer agents, the atypical antipsychotics, which have a somewhat different mechanism of action.

Types of Antipsychotics

The older medications traditionally have been divided into high-potency and low-potency types. They all work basically the same way, but each type has a significantly different side-effect profile.

The high-potency medications, such as haloperidol, require lower doses and produce less sedation. However, they have more of a tendency to produce extrapyramidal (neurological) side effects, such as Parkinsonian-like behavior (tremors, lack of facial expressions, stiff gait).

One problem with the older medications is that they tend to work very well for the positive symptoms of schizophrenia but they often have little or no effect on negative symptoms. This has meant that although the floridly psychotic symptoms were controlled, so that schizophrenics could function outside of hospital settings, they often continued to feel listless, be very isolative, and lead very restricted lives. The newer, atypical agents may help treat the negative symptoms, as well as the positive ones, so that people not only think better, they may also feel better, e.g., they may experience more vitality and a greater sense of "aliveness."

Medication Treatment: What to Expect

Once the diagnosis of schizophrenia or schizophreniform disorder has been made, the physician will probably recommend treatment with an antipsychotic medication. Average doses are shown below.

Dosages of Antipsychotic Medications

Generic Name	Brand Name	Dosage Range (mg/day)	Equiva- lence[1] (mg)
Low Potency			
Chlorpromazine	Thorazine	50–1500	100
Thioridazine	Mellaril	150–800	100
Clozapine[3]	Clozaril	300–900	50
Mesoridazine	Serentil	50–500	50
Quetiapine[3]	Seroquel	300–750	50

High Potency

Molindone	Moban	20–225	10
Perphenazine	Trilafon	8–60	10
Loxapine	Loxitane	50–250	10
Trifluoperazine	Stelazine	10–40	5
Fluphenazine	Prolixin[2]	3–45	2
Thiothixene	Navane	10–60	5
Haloperidol	Haldol[2]	2–40	2
Pimozide	Orap	1–10	1
Risperidone[3]	Risperdal	4–16	1–2
Olanzapine[3]	Zyprexa	5–20	1–2
Sertindole[3]	Serlect	4–24	2
Ziprasidone[3]	Zeldox	80–160	15

Antiparkinson/Anticholinergic Drugs[4]

Trihexyphenidyl	Artane	5–15
Benztropine mesylate	Cogentin	1–8
Biperiden	Akineton	2–8
Amantadine	Symmetrel	100–300

Antipsychotic medications often are initiated in a hospital setting because they can be prescribed more aggressively in the hospital, and high doses are often used. In this chapter, however, the focus is on use in the outpatient setting. From the many possible antipsychotics available, one will be chosen for an initial trial. This choice will be based on the these factors: the previous response to medication, the amount of agitation present, the patient's general health and well-being, including other illnesses, and other medications being taken.

---

1 Dose required to achieve efficacy of 100 mg chlorpromazine.
2 Available in time-release IM formulation.
3 Atypical antipsychotic.
4 Used to treat some antipsychotic side effects.

Based on these and other considerations, a medication will be chosen. Generally, if a particular medication has worked well in the past, it will be used again. If a person is physically healthy and very agitated, a sedating antipsychotic may be chosen. Otherwise, one with fewer sedative and other side effects may be used.

Another decision to be made is whether to use an atypical antipsychotic. Depending on the degree of withdrawal (negative) symptoms, this may be a good first-line choice. Some physicians recommend that atypical antipsychotics should always be used first because of the better response of negative symptoms and the possibility of reduced risk of a particular side effect called tardive dyskinesia (see the section on tardive dyskinesia on page 127). However, atypical antipsychotics don't always work. No one antipsychotic is always effective, nor always well tolerated. Once the medication has been chosen, treatment can be started with a low dose, typically the equivalent of 1 mg of haloperidol two to three times per day (see the chart above).

At the same time that the antipsychotic is started, an anti-Parkinsonian medication (discussed below under "Extrapyramidal Side Effects") is often begun. This second medication is given in order to prevent some possible unpleasant side effects from the antipsychotic medication, such as tremors or muscle spasms.

If there is only a small amount of benefit within a week, the medication can be increased, let's say to the equivalent of 2 mg of haloperidol two to three times per day. It can then be stepped up gradually to an effective dose, or until side effects become a problem. Outside of the hospital, it is unusual to need to go above 20 mg of haloperidol, or the equivalent, per day. And, as stated above, if the first medication does not work, or has intolerable side effects, another medication should be tried.

The choice of the second medication will be based on what was wrong with the first. For example, if the first one was too sedating, a medication that causes less drowsiness will be tried next. Sometimes several medications must be tried before one is found that works and has minimal side effects.

Phases of Treatment

Treatment may be divided into acute and maintenance phases. During the acute phase, medication treatment is initiated and the more prominent psychotic symptoms are controlled. This phase usually lasts from several days to several weeks. Often higher doses of medication are required during the acute phase.

During the maintenance phase, the medication is gradually reduced and more attention is paid to negative symptoms and level of functioning. The maintenance phase is a life-long process in schizophrenia. Thus, involving family members is often important during the maintenance phase for helping the schizophrenic person (or the family members) to recognize the early signs of a recurrence of the illness.

Often, increasing the dosage of the medication can prevent further worsening of the condition. Some of these medications also come in an injectable form that releases the medicine slowly over a period of two to four weeks. This can be very helpful for people who are careless about taking their medications in pill form. With long-term use of the medication, symptoms of tardive dyskinesia (discussed later in this chapter) need to be checked for at least every six months.

Side Effects

Treatment with medication usually involves starting with a low dose of a given medication and gradually raising the dosage until the symptoms are controlled. As the dose is raised, more and more side effects may appear. There are several common types of side effects. If they become intolerable, it is usually helpful to switch to another medication that produces less of that type of side effect. The most common side effects are grouped as follows:

Extrapyramidal Side Effects

This refers to a type of neurological side effects. There are three types of extrapyramidal side effects. They are Parkinsonian, dystonic, and akathisia.

Parkinsonian side effects refer to a group of symptoms that mimic Parkinson's disease. The person's movements are slowed, there may be a tremor, the face shows less expression, and the walk is slow with only small steps possible. *Dystonia* refers to a muscle spasm, usually of the neck. This can be very painful if not treated promptly. *Akathisia* refers to a type of restlessness. The person feels very uncomfortable and cannot sit still. All of these side effects can be treated with anti-Parkinsonian medications (see figure 8.1). By using these medications, higher, more effective, doses of the antipsychotics can be used. The anti-Parkinsonian medications produce side effects of their own, but the dry mouth, blurred vision, and constipation they cause are usually not severe.

Anticholinergic

Antipsychotic medications can cause anticholinergic side effects. These drugs inhibit a part of the nervous system called the cholinergic nervous system and can cause the same side effects as the anti-Parkinsonian medications described above (constipation, dry mouth etc.). Some antipsychotics, like haloperidol, produce very few anticholinergic side effects. Others, like chlorpromazine, produce significant amounts.

Light-Headedness

Antipsychotic medications tend to interfere with the body's ability to maintain a stable blood pressure. Thus, when people taking this kind of medication stand up suddenly from a sitting position, they may experience a brief drop in blood pressure causing light-headedness, which can lead to falls and possible injuries.

Miscellaneous

A multitude of other side effects can be caused by antipsychotic medications. Weight gain is a common one. Antipsychotics tend to interfere with temperature regulation and may lead to heat stroke, especially if the person exercises during warm weather. They also raise prolactin (a hormone) levels and may cause lactation.

Other side effects include Neuroleptic Malignant Syndrome (NMS) a rare, but potentially fatal, reaction to antipsychotic medication. It is characterized by fever, confusion, and rigidity. If not recognized and treated promptly, it can lead to irreversible coma and death.

The medication Clozapine occasionally can cause agranulocytosis, a potentially fatal decrease in the number of white blood cells; therefore, weekly blood tests are required for those taking this medication. And, as with all medications, some people may have allergic reactions. If any of the following side effects is experienced, the doctor should be notified promptly.

- Confusion
- Inability to urinate
- Rash
- Involuntary movements
- Severe sedation
- Prolonged or severe constipation

- Falls
- Muscle spasms
- High fever
- Jaundice
- Severe restlessness

Tardive Dyskinesia

Most of the side effects of antipsychotics appear in the first days or weeks of treatment, but tardive dyskinesia may not appear until after many months or years of treatment. It involves involuntary movements of the face or limbs. Usually, it manifests as twitches of some of the facial muscles. It is of serious concern because there is no really effective treatment and because it may be irreversible, or only very slowly reversible. Thus, antipsychotic medication, unlike the antianxiety and antidepressant medications, can have severe, long-lasting side effects. For this reason, use of the antipsychotics must be approached with more caution. On the other hand, because the psychoses usually are severely debilitating, using these medications may be justified, even lifesaving. When choosing to use these medications, the potential hazards of not treating, e.g., institutionalization, disability, and suicide, must be weighed against the possible side effects.

Are Antipsychotic Medications Habit-Forming?

Antipsychotic medications are definitely not addictive. As a rule, these medications are mildly or moderately unpleasant to take. It is rare to find someone who likes taking them, because there is no "high." People take them because they can function so much better, and because psychosis is so much worse. Even though the medications are not addictive, they do have some potential risks for long-term use, as described above.

Other Treatment Considerations

What if several medications are tried and none works? One important strategy is to reevaluate the diagnosis. For example, is there some type of medical problem contributing to the psychosis?

If the diagnosis is certain, there are other medications that may help. The most likely are the mood stabilizers, the anticonvulsants, and lithium (see chapter 6). Adding one of these to the antipsychotic may be helpful. Sometimes, antianxiety or antidepressant medication may be helpful.

Miscellaneous Disorders

Introduction

In this chapter, we will discuss several types of disorders that generally are less common than those previously discussed, and about which less is known. Most of the types of treatment have already been described in detail in the appropriate chapter, and will only be outlined here. For example, antidepressants are used to treat several of these disorders, and detailed discussions of these drugs can be found in chapter 5. In this chapter, we will briefly describe sleep disorders, attention deficit disorder, eating disorders, borderline personality disorder, post-traumatic stress disorder, aggression, and dementia.

Sleep Disorders

There are many things that can cause disturbed sleep, but here only those disturbances that are referred to as primary sleep disorders will be discussed. These include sleep apnea, nocturnal myoclonus and restless legs syndrome. Other types of sleep disorders are termed "secondary" since the sleep problem is secondary to another disorder, such as anxiety or depression.

Diagnosis

- *Sleep apnea* is characterized by transient periods of the cessation of breathing, or *apnea*, during sleep. These periods last only a few seconds, but they are enough to cause a partial awakening, and thus disturb sleep. They may occur several hundred times each night. Diagnosis can be made by a polysomnogram, taken during a sleep study where breathing, EEG (electro-encephalo-gram), and other vital signs are monitored during sleep. The main symptom of sleep apnea is daytime fatigue, but it is also often associated with loud snoring. Often the person will be unaware of the apneic episodes, and is only aware of being tired all the time.

- *Nocturnal myoclonus* involves sudden jerking movements of the arms and legs during sleep. It also results in daytime fatigue and is diagnosed by polysomnography.

- *Restless Leg Syndrome* involves, as the name suggests, movements and restlessness of the legs that interfere with sleep. It, too, results in fatigue and can be diagnosed by polysomnography.

Sleep Disorders and the Brain

The cause of primary sleep disorders is not fully understood. Sleep apnea can be caused either by the collapse of the muscles of the throat during sleep (obstructive type) and/or by the failure of the respiratory center in the brain to instruct the lungs to breathe during sleep (central type).

Medical Treatment

Generally, sleep apnea is treated with a CPAP (breathing) machine or surgically (tracheostomy). These treatments are fairly effective for treating obstructive apnea, but they are of little bene-fit in central apnea. Nocturnal myoclonus and Restless Legs Syn-drome are treated with medications. Dopaminergic medications, such as bromocriptine, which increase the activity of the neuro-transmitter dopamine, or clonazepam, which is a sedative, can also be effective in treating these problems.

Attention Deficit Disorder

Attention deficit disorder (ADD) is characterized by the inability to focus and sustain one's attention on activities. This disorder begins in early childhood and results in poor school performance and, sometimes, in behavioral problems. A range of 50 to 70 percent of those who develop ADD in childhood will continue to have these problems into adulthood (Hill and Schoener 1996). This results in poor work performance and relationship difficulties. People with ADD are easily bored and find it difficult to focus on a task long enough to complete it. Thus, they fail to complete many tasks and frequently get into trouble for not doing better. They also may seek stimulation, and, as a result, get into trouble for their efforts. Often anxiety and depression develop as a result of these difficulties and low self-esteem is almost always a consequence.

Diagnosis

The diagnosis of ADD is made when people demonstrate difficulty maintaining focused attention on activities. When hyperactivity accompanies ADD, the diagnosis of attention-deficit/hyperactivity disorder (ADHD) is made. This disorder *always* begins in childhood.

Recently, this diagnosis has become somewhat controversial as it is sometimes difficult to diagnose precisely what degree of attentional problems is normal, or what may be caused by situational factors, anxiety, or depression. When six of the following symptoms of inattention have been present for at least six months, ADD can be diagnosed with a fair measure of accuracy:

• Carelessness • Difficulty sustaining attention • Inattentive listening • Failure to follow through on tasks • Difficulty with organizing activities • Avoidance of activities requiring prolonged mental effort • Forgetfulness • Frequent distraction • Frequent loss of materials required for activities

Hyperactivity is diagnosed in children when at least four of the following seven symptoms have been observed for at least six months:

• Fidgeting or squirming • Difficulty staying seated in class • Inappropriate activity—running, climbing • Difficulty playing quietly • Answering questions before they have been completely stated • Difficulty waiting for turn

ADD and the Brain

Many theories have been advanced to explain ADD. In the past, it was called Minimal Brain Dysfunction because it was thought that there was some neurological dysfunction of the brain that interfered with the ability to pay attention. Sometimes, neurological abnormalities can be demonstrated, but most of the time none can be found. It has been shown, however, that ADD tends to be inherited, which implies a biological basis. Positive Emission Tomography (PET) brain scans in the prefrontal cortex of those with ADD have demonstrated an area of decreased metabolic activity (Zametkin et al. 1990). Using MRI scans, other studies have shown a difference in brain structure (Castellanos 1994).

Medical Treatments

Several types of medication are helpful in the treatment of ADD. These include stimulants, antidepressants, and clonidine. Stimulants are the most effective form of treatment, but because they can be habit-forming they have been the subject of much controversy. (It must be noted, however, that properly diagnosed and treated children and adolescents *rarely* abuse the prescribed medications.) Also, many people are reluctant to give psychiatric medication to children, and view it as a form of chemical mind-control. Certainly no one wants to prescribe psychoactive medication for children unless it is absolutely necessary, but the cost of not treating ADD can be high.

When ADD is not treated, children can develop long-lasting psychological problems related to getting into trouble frequently, having adults angry with them often, and being unable to complete many tasks successfully. These experiences can lead to their seeing themselves as "bad" and "failures." These same type of issues arise for adults with ADD who go untreated. Occasionally, some people with ADD are bright enough to get through childhood despite their attentional deficit with few noticeable problems. Then, as adolescents or adults, they begin to have very significant problems.

Treatment Considerations: What to Expect

Treatment is begun with a low dose of medication, such as 5 mg of Ritalin or Dexedrine two to three times a day. If full benefit is not achieved, the dose is gradually increased. Benefit should be noticeable virtually with the first dose, but it may take several days or weeks to evaluate fully. If the child demonstrates excessive nervousness, the dosage should be decreased. If one stimulant does not work, another one can be tried. These medications come in slow-release (SR) forms because the standard preparations may work for only three to four hours, necessitating several doses per day. The more common side effects include anxiety, nervousness, appetite suppression, and insomnia. Usually, these side effects can be controlled by adjusting the amount and timing of the doses.

Antidepressants may also be used. These may be tried initially, in cases where the person has a history of stimulant abuse, or after the stimulants have failed to work. These medications offer the advantage of not being habit-forming, but they have more side effects than the stimulants. Again, it is usual to start with a low dose, and gradually increase the dose until an effective dose is reached. Benefit usually takes two weeks or more to appear. See chapter 5 for a more complete discussion of antidepressants.

Clonidine, normally used to treat high blood pressure, is another medication that is used to treat ADD. It also has some antianxiety properties that can be helpful in treating ADD. It is usually used in combination with other medications. Again one starts with a low dose, usually 0.1 mg, which increases gradually. Typical side effects include low blood pressure (which may cause dizziness) and fatigue or low energy. Other medications, such as antianxiety, antipsychotic, lithium, or anticonvulsant medication may be added to clonidine to gain further benefit. The choice of other medication depends on the presence of other features; for example, someone with ADD who also has mood swings might be treated with a mood stabilizer such as lithium.

Are Stimulants Safe for Long-Term Use?

As with any potentially habit-forming medication, stimulants must be used with caution. Often people get used to the medication so that the dose needs to be increased once or twice. In children, in rare instances, stimulants can cause delayed growth, but this is almost always temporary, and the loss is eventually recovered. These medications have been used for decades without any demonstrable ill effects, and are considered safe for long-term use. A small percentage of people, usually those with a history of drug abuse or with blood relatives who have a history of substance abuse, tend to abuse stimulants, and are best treated with other types of medication (e.g., antidepressants).

Eating Disorders

There are two main types of eating disorders: anorexia and bulimia. Anorexia involves severe weight loss and maintenance of low body weight by restricting food intake, and/or purging (vomiting immediately after eating). People with anorexia are obsessed with their weight and see themselves as fat, despite the fact that they weigh far less than what would be a normal body weight. People with bulimia overeat in binges and then purge after eating. They may consume huge amounts of food and then spend hours purging to avoid gaining weight. They are often slightly overweight.

Diagnosis

The diagnosis of *anorexia* depends on the maintenance of an abnormally low body weight (less than 85 percent of the ideal weight) and a distortion of body image. (No matter how thin anorexics are, they see themselves as fat.) Often they do excessive amounts of exercising to maintain their low weight and they may also use laxatives for purging. Anorexia can lead to severe malnutrition, which can be life-threatening, and always warrants treatment. The diagnosis of *bulimia* depends on frequent binge eating followed by efforts to get rid of the food, either by vomiting, or taking laxatives or diuretics. Bulimia, too, can cause serious medical problems, such as bleeding from a tear in the stomach, or teeth and gum disease.

Eating Disorders and Biology

The cause of eating disorders is not fully understood. Some evidence suggests that anorexia has an addictive aspect. It has been demonstrated that fasting causes the release of endorphins in the brain. These are the brain's own morphine-like substances, which are also released by strenuous exercise. When endorphins are released, they give the person a sense of feeling good, or "high." Thus, it is thought that people with anorexia are, essentially, *addicted* to fasting. Often, anorexia begins when people experience a significant, unintentional, weight loss, from an illness, for example. They then may feel a need to maintain the reduced weight, and to feel very fat if they gain any weight. Then, they take the necessary steps to keep their weight down: restricting their food intake and increasing their exercise.

Bulimia appears to be related to depression. Often people with bulimia engage in binge eating when they are upset, or when they feel emotionally out of control. After bingeing they panic and do something, like inducing vomiting, to get rid of the food.

Medical Treatment

No medication has demonstrated great success in the treatment of anorexia, although several kinds have sometimes been helpful. The most important treatment is weight gain. This is accomplished with a behavioral program that rewards eating and weight gain. With prolonged fasting, the stomach loses its ability to handle food easily. Sometimes medication is used to help the stomach work properly, e.g., cisapride (one brand-name for this drug is Propulsid). Medication like naltrexone, which blocks the "high" of fasting, can be helpful. Naltrexone blocks the effects of opiates and is used to treat heroin addiction and alcoholism. Other types of medication that may be helpful in selected cases include antianxiety, antidepressant, antipsychotic, anticonvulsant medications, and lithium. Bulimia, on the other hand, has been shown to respond well to antidepressants.

Caution: Buproprion (Wellbutrin) cannot be used in the treatment of eating disorders, because of the risk of seizures in this group of patients, but any other antidepressant may be used. Usually an SSRI is used, with good benefit. Sometimes higher doses are required to treat bulimia than are used with depression(e.g. 60 to 80 mg of fluoxetine). Otherwise, treatment with these medications is the same as when they are used to treat depression.

Borderline Personality Disorders

The term "borderline personality disorder" refers to a rather heterogeneous group of disorders. At times, this group has seemed so heterogeneous that the very concept of the diagnosis has been questioned. Originally the term referred to people whose disorder was on the "borderline" between neurosis and psychosis. Over time it has become more refined, but it still retains this association.

Today, the term refers to people whose emotional disorder is more severe than is usually seen in a neurosis, but they are not psychotic, or only transiently so. Studies suggest that about 2 percent of the general population has this disorder, and 10–25 percent of those who are treated in outpatient mental health clinics. Because of their very intense symptomatology they tend to be conspicuous. Their intensely volatile relationships often lead them into legal difficulties and attract the attention of the police, friends, and neighbors.

Diagnosis

In the *Diagnostic and Statistical Manual of Mental Disorders* (DSM-IV) the diagnosis is made by the symptomatology. The following symptoms are the criteria:

- Frantic efforts to avoid abandonment
- Unstable and intense relationships
- Persistently unstable self-image
- Impulsive behavior that is potentially dangerous
- Suicidal or self-mutilating behavior
- Mood swings
- Chronic feelings of emptiness
- Poorly controlled outbursts of anger
- Transient paranoia or dissociative spells

Five of these nine criteria must be present for a diagnosis of borderline personality disorder to be made.

Causes of Borderline Personality Disorder

Many of the writings on borderline personality disorder focus either on traumatic events during childhood, or on the failure of the parents to help the child develop a sturdy sense of self. Other studies look at in-born temperamental factors (Mahler 1975;

Gunderson 1984; Hartocollis 1977; Silver 1992). At the present time there is no definitive answer as to the cause. It would appear that people with borderline personality disorder have a combination of psychological and constitutional factors, in varying degrees.

Medical Treatment

No medication is specific for the treatment of borderline personality disorder, but a number of medication types may help in reducing the symptoms. At the heart of this disorder there is a tendency for intense emotional reactivity or sensitivity to rejection or threat of abandonment. Several kinds of antidepressants, particularly the MAO-inhibitors and SSRIs, can be helpful in reducing this sensitivity to rejection or abandonment (Norden 1989a; 1989; 1995).

Mood stabilizers, including lithium and anticonvulsants, can be helpful in reducing mood swings and controlling anger. Antidepressants can be helpful in treating associated depression and anxiety. Antipsychotic medications can be helpful with paranoia or during periods of disorganization.

Caution: Because of the borderline person's tendency to engage in self-harming behavior, caution must be used when prescribing any medication. It is safest to use only medications that are not likely to be toxic in overdose, and to avoid medications such as the minor tranquilizers, which are habit-forming.

Psychotherapy

Long-term psychotherapy is an important, if not essential, part of the treatment of borderline personality disorder. A good relationship with a therapist can have a very stabilizing effect, and can help the person weather the ups and downs of other relationships. One of the issues that must be addressed is how to handle crises. The borderline person may tend to behave self-destructively in a crisis. Constructive ways of handling the inevitable crises must be explored and reinforced. These include turning to supportive friends, and using crisis hot lines and emergency rooms, and so forth. Some studies show that certain types of group therapy and educational groups can also be very helpful in learning new coping skills (Linehan 1993). See *Shorter-Term Treatment for Borderline Personality Disorders* (Preston 1997) and *I Hate You—Don't Leave Me* (Kreisman 1989) for more complete discussions of this disorder.

Post-Traumatic Stress Disorder

Post-Traumatic Stress Disorder, or PTSD, refers to a set of specific types of reactions to an extremely stressful event. The term PTSD is relatively new. It came into use during the treatment of Vietnam veterans, but the syndrome has been recognized for decades and has variously been called "combat neurosis," "shell shock," or "traumatic" neurosis.

Recently, Post-Traumatic Stress Disorder has become a somewhat controversial diagnosis because in some cases it has been used to apply for disability payments and for damages in litigation; nevertheless it remains an important psychological disorder, with treatments and therapies directed toward the specific set of trauma reactions. Post-Traumatic Stress Disorder is often caused by a combination of exposure to violence and helplessness. For example, children who are physically or sexually abused, or who witnessed spousal abuse would be likely to suffer from PTSD. Adults who were victims of or witness to violent crimes, survivors of natural disasters like earthquakes and floods, and refugees and combatants from war have often been diagnosed with PTSD after the crime or the war ended . It would seem that as violence becomes more commonplace in our modern world, so too the incidence of PTSD increases.

Diagnosis

When people are exposed to a traumatic event, they go through several stages of emotional response.

Initially, there is shock. The person is both horrified and numb. This may last for several hours to several days. Then the person goes through a period of alternating between being overwhelmed with memories of the event and/or being in a state of numbness or emotional detachment. The traumatic memories may come as intrusive images, or flashbacks, or in nightmares. The person feels on edge and is easily startled. There may be intense anxiety, panic attacks and/or depression. Following are the key symptoms of PTSD:

- Increased autonomic arousal, e.g., anxiety, tension, irritability, easily startled, easily overwhelmed by feelings
- Persistent reliving of the trauma (intrusive memories, thoughts, and nightmares)
- Avoidance (social withdrawal and avoidance of any situation that might serve as a reminder of the traumatic event)
- Emotional numbing
- Depression, panic attacks, or substance abuse may also develop as associated features

With emotional support and therapy, over time, most people are gradually able to reestablish a sense of security and to work through most of their feelings about the trauma. However, if the trauma was severe, or took place in childhood, these symptoms may be very persistent.

Medication Treatment

The use of medication in the treatment of PTSD is mostly directed at associated features, such as panic attacks. However, medication is also often used in the initial stage, immediately after the trauma, when the person is feeling very anxious and overwhelmed and having difficulty sleeping. At this time, minor tranquilizers are often used. However, there is some evidence suggesting that minor tranquilizers may interfere with the emotional healing process. Beta blockers may be better for reducing the tension and hypervigilance that are present during the first few days. Then, minor tranquilizers can be used cautiously. SSRIs are being used successfully to reduce overwhelming intrusive symptoms (e.g., flashbacks). If panic attacks, depression, or psychotic symptoms develop, they can be treated with the appropriate medications (as they would when PTSD is not present).

Nonmedication Treatment

Nonmedication forms of treatment are very important in PTSD. In the initial stage some type of crisis debriefing is very helpful for reducing long-term effects. This involves combining some discussion of the actual event, i.e., what exactly happened, with descriptions and explanations of common reactions to such an event, and a great deal of emotional support.

Debriefing is especially helpful when done in a group, such as when many people have been exposed to the same trauma. People tend to fixate about what they could have done differently, and debriefing can help reduce this kind of self-recrimination. Experiencing intense trauma is a major assault on people's sense of being in control of their lives. Reestablishing a sense of control and a feeling of safety is a crucial first step for healing to take place. Ongoing support groups are helpful in diminishing the emotional reactions over time. There are number of support groups organized around specific types of trauma, such as Vietnam veterans, victims of violent crime, and survivors of incest or rape.

Aggression

Aggression, including irritability, hostility, or violent behavior, can be a symptom associated with several mental disorders. It can occur in a number of contexts. When treating aggression it is important to first treat any underlying condition. For example, aggression is fairly common in alcoholism, bipolar disorder, and psychosis. In order to control the aggression, it is first necessary to control the primary disorder. These are the disorders that are frequently associated with aggression: Attention Deficit Disorder, Antisocial Personality Disorder, Borderline Personality Disorder, Conduct Disorder, Delirium, Dementia, Depression, Intermittent Explosive Disorder (sudden episodes of aggressive behavior), Medication-induced aggression, Mania (Bipolar Disorder), Mental retardation, Paranoid Disorder, Postconcussion Syndrome (following brain trauma or head injury), Schizophrenia, Substance Use Disorders, and Temporal Lobe Epilepsy.

As stated above, quite often the aggression can be controlled by treating the primary disorder. For example, those suffering from paranoid psychosis may become violent because they think people are trying to kill them. When the psychosis is treated and they are no longer paranoid, the tendency toward violence usually subsides. Sometimes medications are used more specifically to try to control the aggression. Medications that may be helpful include anticonvulsants, antipsychotics, beta blockers, buspirone, clonidine, lithium, and SSRIs. The choice of medication is guided by the presence of associated features. For example, a person with aggression associated with mood swings might be treated with a mood stabilizer, such as lithium or an anticonvulsant, such as valproate. The following list shows which types of medication target specific associated features of various disorders.

Medication Types	Associated Features/Disorders
Anticonvulsants (e.g., carbamazepine)	Labile mood, poor impulse control, organicity (some kind of damage to the brain)
Antipsychotics	Disorganized behavior
Beta blockers (e.g., Propranolol)	Organicity (e.g., dementia)
Buspirone	Organicity
Clonidine	Anxiety, agitation
Lithium	Labile mood, impulsivity
SSRIs	Anger "attacks"

Dementia

Dementia refers to a condition in which there is a significant impairment in cognitive functioning, especially memory. Alzheimer's disease is the most well-known type of dementia, but other types are fairly common, too. These include Pick's disease, multi-infarct dementia, Parkinson's disease, and alcoholic dementia. Dementia is not caused by aging, but it does tend to become more common as people grow older. Approximately 10 percent of the population have dementia and/or significant memory impairment at age seventy, 20 percent at age eighty (APA 1989), and 80 percent at age ninety. When evaluating dementia, a thorough medical evaluation is crucial, including laboratory tests, to look for diseases that cause dementia, and often a brain scan, as well. Some studies indicate that about 15 percent of those diagnosed with dementia illness have treatable medical conditions, which, if treated, might cure the dementia (APA 1989).

Medical Treatment

New medications are being developed for the treatment of Alzheimer's disease. Tacrine (Cognex) was the first, but it can have significant liver toxicity and requires multiple doses per day. A newer medication, donepezil (Aricept), avoids these problems. These medications do not cure Alzheimer's disease, but can sometimes improve alertness and cognitive functioning in people who are in the early stage of the disease (i.e., in terms of mental functioning, often they can effectively roll back the clock for about one year for Alzheimer's patients). Their usefulness in other types of dementia is under study. Other medications are in development.

Other types of dementia are helped by treating the underlying cause, whenever possible. Even when the dementia itself is not treatable, different aspects of the disorder may be treatable. For example, people who have dementia often become paranoid because they do not understand what is going on around them. Antipsychotic medication is usually effective for treating this. Agitation and depression are sometimes seen in those with dementia and may benefit from treatment with antidepressant or antianxiety medication.

10

Medication During Pregnancy, Childhood, Adolescence, and Old Age

Pregnancy and Psychotropic Medications

Some of the most frequently asked questions about psychotropic medications concern their safety if they are taken during pregnancy. However, before specific discussion about particular medications is provided, it is important to explain how information regarding safe drug use during pregnancy is obtained, because there are limits as to how research in this area can be carried out.

How Safety Is Determined

Much of the information about safe use during pregnancy comes from studies done on animals. Although these studies are extensive, it cannot be assumed that the findings necessarily will apply to humans. Even if there are human studies available, they are often not conducted among large numbers of people, so applying the results to the general population must be done cautiously.

Therefore, it may be very difficult for your doctor to give you an absolute answer about whether a particular drug has been shown to be safe.

Some drugs are safer than others during pregnancy, while some other drugs should be avoided entirely. Still others are considered safe only during the second and third trimester and should not be given in the first trimester. Because the first trimester is the period when fetal cells are rapidly growing, dividing, and forming into organs, it is considered the time of highest risk for damage from medicines. However, organs, including the brain, continue to develop during the second and third trimesters and even after birth. Thus, some medicines could be potentially harmful to the baby throughout an entire pregnancy. Furthermore, these effects might be of such a nature that they might not be noticed until later in the child's life; for example, behavioral problems would not be apparent during infancy.

Keep in mind that women often do not realize they are pregnant until after conception has taken place and fetal development has begun. Therefore, before starting a new medication, it is important that your doctor is aware of any plans you may have for becoming pregnant in the near future. In this situation, you and your doctor might have to decide whether this is the best time for you to have a baby, and take into account what would happen if you didn't start a particular medicine right now. Obviously, this is a very personal and complex issue, but it is faced frequently by women who wish to become pregnant and who also may require medications to treat their depression, for example.

Complications of Pregnancy and Medication

A brief summary of the types of complications that are known to occur with medications taken during pregnancy is provided below:

- Teratogenesis—malformation of the fetus or fetal organs (this risk is greatest during the first trimester when organs are being formed)
- Drug effects on the growth and development of the fetus
- Drug effects on labor and delivery
- Residual drug effects on the newborn
- The impact that pregnancy can have on the way a drug works

- Drug effects on the breast-fed infant

Breast-Feeding and Medications

Taking medicines while breast-feeding can be cause for concern. Knowledge in this area has increased dramatically in recent years, however, there are still many unanswered questions. For the most part, when a medicine passes into breast milk, the concentration of the drug has been diluted in comparison to the amount in the mother's bloodstream. So even though the medication may be measurable in breast milk, it may produce no, or minimal, negative effects on the baby. Many medicines, therefore, have a relatively safe track record when taken by nursing mothers.

On the other hand, some medications can produce extreme negative effects on the baby even in small amounts, so their use should be avoided while breast-feeding. An example of such a medication would be cancer chemotherapy agents. Still other medicines reach a high enough concentration in breast milk to be of serious concern. Lithium, for example, is known to reach levels in breast milk equivalent in the baby's bloodstream to about 40 percent of that in the mother's bloodstream, which can lead to the potential for serious harm to the baby. It is strongly recommended that women taking lithium not breast-feed (American Society of Hospital Pharmacists 1996).

The following table is a brief summary, by drug category, of some known information about medications and pregnancy and breast-feeding. If you have any concerns about a specific drug, discuss them thoroughly with your doctor.

Children, Adolescents, and Psychotropic Medications

Children and adolescents are often treated with psychotropic medicines. This practice has sparked a national debate. Some people argue that children do not suffer from "true" mental health problems because their problems are not of a biological nature and that most symptoms can be corrected by a change in environment or parenting style. Those who hold this belief contend that the real causes of emotional distress in children and adolescents are societal pressures and family lifestyle changes, which have led to the emergence of emotional and behavioral problems in children.

Table 10.1   Pregnancy, Breast-Feeding, and Drugs

Class of Medication	Comments	Teratogenicity	Effects on Newborn from Exposure During Pregnancy	Found in Breast Milk
Antidepressants	There is inconclusive data on whether the rate of miscarriages is increased with antidepressants MAOIs and bupropion have not been studied widely in humans	Not established	• For tricyclic antidepressants, effects on the newborn can include drowsiness and difficulty urinating • For serotonin type antidepressants, effects on the newborn can include restlessness and difficulty sleeping	Yes
Antipsychotics	Antipsychotics may be preferred over lithium for bipolar disorder during the first trimester The lowest possible dose is recommended	Not suspected	• Low motor activity	Yes
Anticonvulsants (valproic acid and carbamazepine)		All are known or suspected to be teratogens (producing fetal malformations)	• Suspected risk of spinal bifida	Yes
Lithium	Historically, lithium use has not been advised during pregnancy. However, your doctor might consider lithium safer than anticonvulsants in the second and third trimester—with very close monitoring.	Known	• Possible malformation of heart valve	Yes—to a high degree
Benzodiazepines	Avoid in first trimester	Some are known teratogens	• Low motor activity and drowsiness • Possible drug withdrawal	Yes

On the other hand, those who have witnessed the benefits of medications also present some strong arguments. Seeing a child's self-esteem improve because of better school performance and social adjustment, or witnessing a child come back from the brink of suicide are strong arguments in the opposite direction. Furthermore, there is increasing evidence that genetic influences can predispose a child or teenager to depression, bipolar disorder, or Attention Deficit Disorder (ADD).

Both sides present passionate and convincing arguments. As with most worthy debates, the answers will probably lie somewhere in the middle and incorporate elements of both sides' arguments. Until this complex issue is resolved, however, it is a reality that children are receiving a variety of medicines, most commonly stimulants, antidepressants, and mood stabilizers. It is not the intention of this book to preferentially support either side. Rather, we want to provide you with as much information as possible so that, if medicines are prescribed for your children, their use will lead to a successful outcome.

If a child in your care is taking medicines, or if you are trying to decide whether to begin a medication regimen, there are some steps you can take to ensure the safest and most effective course of treatment. These measures are described below.

Safety Issues for Younger People

Make sure you understand the diagnosis and how it was made. The prescribing of psychiatric medications can be done by general practitioners, pediatricians, or psychiatrists. Ask for a detailed explanation as to why the doctor has decided that a particular medication is necessary, for example, a stimulant, or antidepressant. Find out how often the doctor treats this particular condition. Ideally, the treatment is being provided by a highly trained child or adolescent psychiatrist who has obtained a complete psychological testing profile from a psychologist. However, in reality, many areas of the country are in short supply of mental health professionals. If your primary care doctor or pediatrician is prescribing psychiatric medication for your child, make sure you are comfortable with his or her expertise in the area; that is, does the physician have specialized training in the field as evidenced by his/her licensure? Does the local mental health association recommend the doctor? You could also get a second opinion on the doctor's qualifications. Talk to others—parents and children— being treated for the same condition.

Social Environment Issues

The parent or caregiver of a child who has been prescribed a course of psychiatric medication must understand that medications are probably only a part of the treatment that will be required. As with adults, but in a more complex manner, environmental factors may be contributing to the child's current difficulties. Be aware that some family therapy may need to take place, or that some social factors may need to change. Be willing to participate actively in the complete treatment plan.

Compliance

You must also understand the necessity of compliance. It will be important to identify any barriers to ensuring that the medication is taken consistently. For example, some school systems will not allow medications to be brought to, or stored on, school premises. This can create the need to time doses very carefully so that none are missed.

The child may have multiple residences. You must make sure that there is a supply of medicine at each house. Are there members of the child's family, or school system, who are opposed to the medicine? It is essential to encourage everyone involved in your child's care to honestly discuss what reservations they may have. When family members or caregivers do not support the prescribed treatment, the child receives mixed signals and may become distressed and confused.

Legal Issues

For certain stimulants, special prescriptions are required every time the medicine is filled at a pharmacy. This is federal law and there are no "ways to get around it." The doctor has to write these prescriptions by hand, and they cannot be "refilled" in the traditional sense. This legal requirement can lead to frustration, and more importantly, to missed doses, if careful planning is not done ahead of time. Do not get close to running out of medicine. Know when your doctor's office is open and closed. Find out if your doctor has a colleague or partner who could write a prescription in an emergency.

Dosages for Younger People

When the doctor prescribes a medication for a child or teenager, there are some general dosing considerations that are taken into account. Younger children, especially, may be more sensitive to side effects. It is advisable to start out with a low dose, sometimes a small test dose, and increase the dosage slowly over time. Be sure you understand exactly what the dosing range is for the medicine your child is taking. Sometimes dosages are based on your child's weight. Make sure your doctor is aware of any changes in your child's weight.

It is generally assumed that children are more efficient metabolizers of medication than adults and even adolescents. Therefore, the amount of medication in the bloodstream might be more susceptible to ups and downs. Sometimes, a medicine that an adult can take on a once-a-day basis may need to be given two or three times a day to a child.

Children are susceptible to the full range of side effects from any given medication. Some side effects may be of greater concern. For example, the cardiac side effects of tricyclic antidepressants may be more serious in children than in adults. It is also necessary to take some special precautions if your child is receiving a tricyclic antidepressant. Be sure to ask your doctor about the safe use of tricyclics for your child.

To summarize, psychiatric medications can be a safe and effective part of your child's treatment. It is very likely, however, that medicine will not be all that is required to help your child get better. Learning as much as possible about the medicine and finding a qualified doctor to work with will greatly increase the chances of successful treatment.

The Elderly

The aging process is associated with the appearance of multiple medical conditions, most of which most likely will be treated with one or more medications. This can result in the risk of serious drug-drug interactions. To avoid such complications, it is essential the doctor has a full medical history and a complete list of current medicines.

In the past, certain mental health conditions were often not identified and treated in the elderly. That trend has changed. For example, it has become apparent that depression is not a normal part of aging and that the elderly do not have to suffer with untreated depression. Consequently, the aged population is more likely than ever to be receiving a psychiatric medication. When these are combined with medicines for physical illness, the chance of unintended drug interactions further increases.

Another problem associated with aging is the difficult time many people have in adhering to their prescribed medicines. Forgetfulness is sometimes the reason, especially for those who live alone. Many other causes have been identified, such as incomplete understanding of the medicine, impaired vision or hearing, or purposely taking less to avoid side effects. Limited or fixed incomes may mean that elderly people cannot pay for their medication regularly, causing intermittent compliance.

Furthermore, many biological systems change as a result of aging. Decreases in kidney and liver function are expected in the elderly. These changes increase the chance that medications can accumulate to seriously high levels in the body. Total body fat increases with age, which affects how some drugs are stored in the body (see chapter 4 for a discussion of drug distribution within the body). Also, older people sometimes neglect their nutritional and fluid requirements. Being undernourished or dehydrated can create problems for people taking certain medications, such as lithium.

Neurotransmitter systems are likely to change as a result of aging. This means that older people have different responses to a given drug than younger people do. Usually, the change is in the direction of increased sensitivity to the medicine, which can mean that the average adult dose is likely to be too much for an older person. Extreme sensitivity to side effects occurs in the elderly. The side effects listed below are of particular concern for older people who are taking psychiatric medications:

Side Effects in the Elderly

- Changes in mental functioning—impaired memory, decreased alertness, confusion, lethargy, slowed reaction times
- Changes in heart rate and blood pressure—a drop in blood pressure can lead to light-headedness and dizziness with an end result of falls and fractures. Other factors can combine to further increase the risk of fall, for instance, arthritic conditions

that impede mobility and balance, or nighttime awakening with disorientation.

- Drying effects—constipation, dry mouth, blurred vision, urinary retention
- Movement disorders—pacing, rigid arms and legs, problems with walking

Most medical practitioners are aware of the general steps that can be taken to minimize some of the difficulties described above. In addition, the following precautions should be observed:

- Nonmedication treatments should be considered and maximized
- Dosages generally should be reduced
- More medicines than are necessary should be avoided
- Side effects should be recognized and treated promptly
- If problems arise, they should be communicated immediately to a health care provider

In recent years, many articles have been published about the aging population. Not only is the percentage of people sixty-five-years and older increasing, but the number of the "old-old" (over eighty-five-years-old) is also increasing. The challenges associated with adequate medical and psychiatric treatment of this age group will be great. There is, however, good cause for optimism. Today, geriatric medicine and geriatric psychiatry are established specialty areas. Undoubtedly, increasing research and attention to this age group will result in more comprehensive and compassionate care.

11

Nonpharmaceutical Approaches

Many people suffering from psychological symptoms may choose not to be treated with psychiatric medications, even if they have a disorder that would be medication-responsive. There are a number of reasons that this may be the case. Topping the list are concerns regarding the safety of psychotropic medications. Although many of these drugs, as mentioned in previous chapters, are safe, the fact remains that all medications do have some side effects; this is an understandable concern. A second reason is that some people, arc allergic to or intolerant of various psychiatric medications and for those reasons are unable to take them. A third reason is cost. Many of the older generation medications are currently available in generic form, and the cost is minimal. However, most of these medications, as mentioned in earlier chapters, have significantly more side effects. Newer medications that are better tolerated and less toxic are often rather expensive. For example, some people being treated with the newer antidepressants may have to pay between one and four dollars per day. This can be a financial hardship for some people, particularly those who live on fixed incomes. Finally, of course, there is the matter of personal choice, as some folks simply prefer using nonmedical approaches for combating psychological problems (e.g., psychotherapy).

Many of the approaches addressed in this chapter can be used as adjuncts to medication treatment and/or psychotherapy.

In fact, several of these approaches are strongly recommended because of their track record of effectiveness in enhancing psychological wellness (especially physical exercise and techniques designed to improve sleep).

Sleep: The Royal Road to Mental Health

If one could identify the single most common stress symptom, seen in almost all types of psychiatric disorders, it would be sleep disturbance. Sleep is an incredibly important biological function. It is essential to restoring and maintaining both emotional and physical health. However, it is quite fragile and prone to disruption by a host of factors. In the past three decades a significant amount of research has been accomplished in an attempt to understand more about sleep. Though much has been learned, there still exist a number of mysteries about the function of sleep.

What is clearly known is that sleep deprivation does a lot more than simply contribute to daytime drowsiness. With even a couple of nights of significantly disrupted sleep, most people will experience noticeable problems in thinking (in particular, an impaired ability to maintain attention and concentration); most also will show signs of decreased emotional control. Sleep deprivation dramatically alters brain chemistry. Presumably, the ability of certain brain areas to regulate emotions becomes compromised; the result is increased emotional sensitivity, poor tolerance for frustration, and stronger emotional reactions (e.g., tearfulness or irritability). Thus, almost all psychiatric disorders are made a lot worse by the presence of a sleep disturbance. In addition, even a couple of nights of very poor sleep have been shown to have an adverse impact on the immune system, and may be responsible for increased risk of infectious illnesses (such as colds or the flu). And of course, there is daytime fatigue and drowsiness.

One of the most helpful things a person can do when experiencing any type of emotional distress is to improve the quality of sleep. When we suggest this to our clients, they often dismiss the advice. It seems like a trivial concern to them, especially when compared to the serious life events that are currently plaguing them. But we want to underscore how much disturbed sleep can contribute to emotional suffering, and, conversely, how much enhanced sleep can be a direct way to improve emotional functioning.

Sleep Enhancement

The following behaviors have been shown to be very helpful for enhancing sleep:

- Do not drink beverages that contain caffeine. It is important to note that many drinks do contain caffeine, not just coffee. Also, many people report that they drink caffeine only in the morning, and not later in the day. However, be aware that even if ingested only in the morning, and even if there is no difficulty going to sleep, any amount of caffeine may result in sleep that is (1) more restless, and (2) less deep (that is, there is reduced time spent in stages 3 and 4 sleep, which are the stages in which deep sleep occurs). A very common habit pattern is to drink moderate to heavy amounts of caffeine during the day, fail to get adequate deep sleep at night, and then to awaken the next day feeling very tired. Then, guess what?—the person drinks more caffeine to ward off drowsiness.

- Avoid emotionally intense experiences prior to retiring to bed (this includes arguments with your spouse or even action-packed movies). These experiences always generate the release of stress hormones that interfere with the ability to go to sleep.

- Use the bed for only two activities: sleeping and love making.

- Turn down the lights about one-half hour before retiring. The brain is programmed to respond chemically to environmental cues, one of which is light. As light levels decrease, activating neurotransmitters shut down, and certain brain chemicals (i.e., melatonin) are secreted, lowering arousal levels in the brain and making the transition to sleep easier.

- Immersion in hot water, gentle stretches, and relaxation exercises are tried and true approaches to improve sleep. Muscle tension sends nerve impulses up the spinal cord and keeps the brain in a state of excitation. For this reason, any number of activities that result in decreased muscle tension can help improve the ability to fall asleep.

- Avoid the use of alcohol. Although alcohol may cause relaxation and drowsiness, it can also interfere with sleep. In particular, as the alcohol is being metabolized by the body, it is chemically altered. Several hours after drinking alcohol some of these metabolic by-products actually stimulate the brain and cause the person either to wake up (in the middle of the night) or to enter into only the lightest stages of sleep.

- Reduce worry. Of course this is a lot easier said than done! However, ongoing thinking and worrying about troublesome matters late in the evening has a way of keeping the brain in a state of excitation. This may explain why counting sheep sometimes works to put people to sleep. With the mind focused on sheep, it won't be attending to worries. Plus, it is pretty damned boring to watch sheep jump over a fence. This form of mental activity is not at all likely to stimulate most people.

- Engage in regular exercise. Exercise has many benefits but when it comes to sleep, it has demonstrated a powerful ability to yield significantly better quality sleep (especially increased time spent in deep sleep). How much exercise and what kind? It is hard to know for sure, but the indications are that aerobic exercise is best, although less strenuous exercise can also be helpful. Also, 20 minutes, three times a week seems to be adequate, although most experts recommend at least some exercise each day. **Note:** It is important to note that strenuous exercise should *not* take place in the two hours just prior to retiring. Exercise before bedtime actually can interfere with sleep, thus you should plan to exercise earlier in the day.

- Reset your biological clock and enhance your sleep. This can be accomplished by two activities. The first is to establish highly regular times for going to sleep and awakening. Biological systems and rhythms have been observed to organize around these predictable cycles. A second strategy is to get early morning bright light exposure (upon awakening, be sure to open the blinds and let the sunshine in, or in winter months, go to a very well-lighted place in your home for the first 30 minutes of the morning). This early morning bright light exposure is believed to recalibrate the circadian rhythm, which plays an important role in regulating brain chemistry in general, and in influencing sleep patterns in particular.

Influencing Serotonin Levels in the Brain

In previous chapters we discussed the role of serotonin and its influence in various emotional disorders (e.g., depression, obsessive compulsive disorder (OCD), and panic disorder). As you may have noticed, serotonin has also received a good deal of media attention. What's all the hype about serotonin?

Serotonin appears to be a sort of multipurpose stabilizing neurotransmitter. It functions in many parts of the brain to inhibit neuron firing, and, in a sense, it acts as a braking mechanism, helping to regulate the internal chemical environment of the brain. In humans and other mammals, if serotonin levels are increased, aggression and irritability decrease. If serotonin is increased, it also decreases the likelihood of panic attacks. Furthermore, people suffering from major depression often recover when their serotonin levels are increased.

Certainly, one way to increase serotonin activity in the brain is to take antidepressants that have an impact on the serotonin system (i.e., the SSRIs, such as Prozac or Paxil). There may be nonpharmacologic ways of increasing serotonin, too. Some research supports the notion that the following activities may result in an increase in serotonin (Norden 1995):

- Exposure to bright light.

- Repetitive muscular movements. This may include such diverse activities as walking, knitting, chewing gum, or rocking in a rocking chair. (Isn't it interesting how these activities are often experienced as relaxing or soothing? Have you ever wondered why rocking a crying baby can be so calming?)

- Strenuous physical exercise

- Eating a snack that contains complex carbohydrates (such as whole grain bread). This may help to facilitate the absorption of amino acids into the brain, which is necessary for the production of neurotransmitters like serotonin.

- Crying *may* increase serotonin, although this is just speculation.

- Experiencing mastery. Studies with monkeys have shown that if a new monkey is introduced into an established troop of monkeys, initially, its serotonin levels will be either in the average range or somewhat below average. However, if this monkey establishes dominance and succeeds in becoming the dominant monkey, its serotonin levels increase. Similarly, serotonin levels measured in college students have been found to be higher in those who were leaders or excelled in athletics. There is, of course, an interesting question here: what comes first; dominance and mastery or high serotonin levels? Current speculation holds that it can go either way: those with already high serotonin may be more likely to succeed; however, it may also be that as people—or monkeys, for that matter—learn and practice how to be more assertive, powerful, or effective, that these experiences may affect the brain by increasing serotonin levels.

"Health Foods" and Herbs

For a number of years, vitamins, minerals, and other food supplements have been advocated as treatments for psychiatric symptoms. These recommendations were derived from the knowledge that many important brain chemicals (that is, neurotransmitters such as serotonin and norepinephrine) are produced in the brain and use amino acids as their chemical building blocks.

Also, it has been discovered that some fairly rare psychiatric disorders can be caused by severe vitamin deficiencies (one example is Korsakoff's Syndrome, which is most commonly seen in people with a history of severe alcoholism who suffer from malnutrition and vitamin B-1 deficiency). In the 1960s and 1970s, there was great hope that psychiatric disorders could be helped by treatment with megadoses of vitamins and improved diets. The results, however, have been disappointing. Such approaches aimed at treating schizophrenia and major depression have failed to produce the desired effects, and have been successful only in the cases of Korsakoff's Syndrome and other very rare diseases.

Although amino acids (such as tyrosine and tryptophan) and vitamins *are* important for the healthy functioning of the brain, it appears that almost everyone who eats a reasonably healthy diet receives ample supplies of these essential chemicals. Furthermore, even though a person might ingest large amounts of these supplements, these molecules have only a very limited capacity to enter the brain, and thus have little if any impact on brain functioning. At times, very high doses of vitamins have produced serious side effects and toxicity.

Typically, health food supplements are rarely subjected to carefully controlled research, and, in most instances, reports of "successful treatment" with vitamins and amino acids are only anecdotal and not substantiated by scientific research. Because most of these products are not regulated by the Food and Drug Administration, their strength and purity vary tremendously, and adequate studies that examine potential drug-drug interactions are rare. (Thus questions remain regarding the safety of these products.) Still, despite the absence of solid research, health food supplements continue to be purchased by people seeking relief from emotional suffering.

Recent times, however, have seen the emergence of two products considered to be "health food supplements" that do appear to have some promise.

Melatonin

Melatonin is a naturally produced hormone that is manufactured in the brain by the pineal gland. It is believed to play a role in regulating the circadian rhythm and sleep cycles in human beings and numerous other animals. It has received a good deal of media attention during the past few years, primarily as a treatment for sleep disorders.

Unlike many other so-called health foods, melatonin has been the subject of numerous research studies in the past twenty-five years. It does appear to have useful applications in the treatment of some sleep disorders (primarily for jet lag and sleep problems caused by changing work-and-sleep schedules as seen in those who are shift workers). It must be stated, however, that the use of melatonin should still be considered experimental, and anyone considering taking this preparation should speak to a physician or pharmacist first. There have been indications that melatonin use may aggravate depression, and thus at this time, it is not advised that it be taken by people who suffer from depression. Finally, there is a significant unknown; it is very unclear how melatonin interacts with other prescription medications. Until more research is done, this hormone should be taken with caution.

St. John's Wort

Another preparation that has been subject to a lot of media attention lately is *St. John's Wort* (the Latin name is hypericum perforatum). This herbal treatment is derived from the flowers of the hypericum plant. It has been used in Germany during the past ten years primarily to treat depression. The precise way that hypericum works is not known, but there is speculation that it increases serotonin levels in the brain. St. John's Wort, unlike most other herbal remedies, has been the subject of a fair amount of research. In a recent review of the literature, it has been shown to be effective in relieving symptoms of depression in those suffering from mild-to-moderate depression (Bloomfield et al. 1996). It has few side effects, and is generally well-tolerated. Reports indicate that the time required to begin to see symptomatic improvement may be longer than that of standard antidepressants (which sometimes require six weeks or more of treatment before the onset of positive effects). The drug, however, does not appear to be effective in treating moderate-to-severe depression, and, at the time of this writing, no long-term treatment studies are available.

St. John's Wort may prove to be a safe and useful approach for treating mild depression, however, it too must be considered an experimental treatment for the time being. Also, drug-drug interactions are not well understood, and most physicians strongly urge that people not take St. John's Wort along with prescription antidepressants because there is the possibility of provoking a potentially serious reaction called a serotonin syndrome.

For more information on St. John's Wort, the reader is referred to Bloomfield et al. *Hypericum and Depression* (1996). Or information can be obtained from the following Internet site: http://www.hypericum.com

One final concern about health foods is that their availability as over-the-counter products can cause people to bypass the critical step of obtaining an accurate and thorough diagnosis from a trained professional. As indicated in several chapters of this book, many psychiatric disorders are best treated by a combination of medication and psychotherapy. The over-the-counter status of these products may lead some people to believe that depression, for instance, can be treated simply by a trip to the health food store. Potentially, psychotherapy could be ignored in favor of "natural" treatment with herbal remedies. The profoundly positive, and often life-changing impact of psychotherapy would be tragically absent from a person's attempts at a complete recovery.

PART II

Guide to Psychiatric Drugs

To the best of our knowledge, recommended doses of medications listed in this book are accurate. However, they are not meant to serve as a guide for the prescribing of medications. Physicians, please check the manufacturer's product information sheet or the *Physicians' Desk Reference* for any changes in dosage schedule or for contraindications.

Warnings and Cautions

Alcohol

Most of the drugs listed in this Guide can cause drowsiness, especially when they are first started. Alcohol can intensify this effect. The stimulants—amphetamine, methylphenidate, and pemoline—do not cause drowsiness, but they can mask some of the effects of alcohol and increase the chance of seizures.

Driving

Most of the drugs listed in this Guide can cause slowed reaction times. The stimulants—amphetamine, methylphenidate, and pemoline—can mask signs of drowsiness or slowed reaction times. In all cases, it is necessary to take care when driving, operating machinery, or doing jobs that require alertness.

Storage

All drugs should be kept in the original container, out of childrens' reach. Drugs should be stored away from direct light, in a cool, dry place. Do not store drugs in the refrigerator unless directed to do so. Discard outdated or expired drugs safely.

Directory of Brand Names

If you want information about a particular medication and you have only the brand name, look at the directory below. Brand names are all listed in the left-hand column. To the right of the brand name, you will see the generic name or a general drug category. Generic names appear in alphabetical order in the pages that follow. First, find the generic name under which the drug will be found. Then, turn to the alphabetized entry.

Brand Name . . . . **Generic Name**

Adapin . . . . doxepin
Adderall. . . . . amphetamine
Amphetamine . . . . amphetamine
Ambien . . . . zolpidem
Anafranil . . . . clomipramine
Artane . . . . trihexyphenidyl
       (see anticholinergics/
       antidyskinetics)
Asendin. . . . . amoxapine
Atarax . . . . hydroxyzine
       (see antihistamines)
Ativan . . . . lorazepam
Aventyl . . . . nortriptyline
Benadryl . . . . diphenhydramine
       (see antihistamines)
BuSpar . . . . busiprone
Catapres. . . . . clonidine
Cibalith-S . . . . lithium
Clozaril . . . . clozapine
Cogentin . . . . benztropine
       (see anticholinergics/
       antidyskinetics)
Corgard . . . . nadolol
       (see beta blockers)
Cylert. . . . . pemoline
Dalmane . . . . flurazepam
Depakene . . . . valproate
Depakote . . . . valproate
Desoxyn. . . . . amphetamine
Desyrel . . . . trazodone

Brand Name	Generic Name
Dexedrine	amphetamine
Dextroamphetamine	amphetamine
Doral	quazepam
Effexor	venlafaxine
Effexor XR	venlafaxine
Elavil	amitriptyline
Eskalith	lithium
Halcion	triazolam
Haldol decanoate	haloperidol
Haldol	haloperidol
Inderal	propanolol (see beta blockers)
Klonopin	clonazepam
Libritabs	chlordiazepoxide
Librium	chlordiazepoxide
Lithobid	lithium
Lithonate	lithium
Lithotabs	lithium
Lopressor	metoprolol (see beta blockers)
Loxitane	loxapine
Ludiomil	maprotiline
Luvox	fluvoxamine
Mellaril	thioridazine
Moban	molindone
Nardil	phenelzine
Navane	thiothixene
Norpramin	desipramine
Orap	pimozide
Pamelor	nortriptyline
Parnate	tranylcypromine
Paxil	paroxetine
Paxipam	halazepam
Permitil	fluphenazine
Prolixin	fluphenazine
ProSom	estazolam
Prozac	fluoxetine
Remeron	mirtazapine

Brand Name . . . .   Generic Name

Restoril . . . . temazepam
Risperdal . . . . risperidone
Ritalin . . . . methylphenidate
Ritalin SR . . . . methylphenidate
Serax . . . . oxazepam
Serentil . . . . mesoridazine
Seroquel. . . . . quetiapine
Serzone . . . . nefazodone
Sinequan . . . . doxepin
Stelazine. . . . . trifluoperazine
Surmontil . . . . trimipramine
Symmetrel . . . . amantadine
        (see anticholinergics/
        antidyskinetics)
Tegretol . . . . carbamazepine
Tegretol XR . . . . carbamazepine
Tenormin . . . . atenolol
        (see beta blockers)
Thorazine . . . . chlorpromazine
Tofranil . . . . imipramine
Tofranil PM . . . . imipramine
Tranxene . . . . clorazepate
Tranxene SD . . . . clorazepate
Trilafon . . . . perphenazine
Valium . . . . diazepam
Valrelease . . . . diazepam
Visken . . . . pindolol
        (see beta blockers)
Vistaril . . . . hydroxyzine
        (see antihistamines)
Vivactil . . . . protriptyline
Wellbutrin SR . . . . bupropion
Wellbutrin. . . . . bupropion
Xanax. . . . . alprazolam
Zoloft. . . . . sertraline
Zyprexa . . . . olanzapine

Drug Name: ALPRAZOLAM   (al-PRAZ-o-lam)

Drug Category: Antianxiety medicine

Requires prescription, controlled substance, moderate potential for abuse

Commonly Used Brand-Name Products
Tablets   Xanax (and generic) 0.25 mg, 0.5 mg, 1 mg, and 2 mg

GENERAL INFORMATION

Highly effective in treating anxiety, nervousness, and panic disorder.

Before Taking this Medication

Talk to your doctor about the benefits and risks associated with alprazolam. Make sure you understand how to take it safely and effectively. You and your family members should be very familiar with the side effects and signs of having too much in your system. Make sure your doctor has the following information in detail:

- any allergic or bad reactions you have had to alprazolam or any other medication
- all prescription and over-the-counter medicines you are taking
- your complete medical history
- if you are pregnant, could be pregnant, or are planning a pregnancy in the near future, alprazolam should not be taken
- if you are breast-feeding, alprazolam can pass into breast milk and could affect the baby

DOSAGE

The starting dose of alprazolam will be low and gradually be increased depending on your response.

Adults:

Anxiety: 0.25 to 0.5 mg up to 3 times a day.

Panic disorder: 0.5 mg to 2 mg up to 4 times a day.

Older adults are more susceptible to side effects and will generally require lower dosages.

Children under 18: Safe use has not been established in this age group.

DIRECTIONS FOR PROPER USE
- *Take exactly as prescribed. Do not take more or less than prescribed. Alprazolam levels that are too high can cause serious toxicity.*
- If you take alprazolam regularly for an extended period of time, do not stop taking it unless told to do so by your doctor. It may be necessary to gradually reduce the dose before stopping completely.
- If you miss a dose, take it as soon as possible. However, if the missed dose is within 4 hours of your next dose, skip the missed dose and resume with your next scheduled dose.

PRECAUTIONS
Alcohol should be avoided while taking alprazolam.

Side Effects
Not all side effects will occur. Many side effects will diminish with time. *However, some side effects may be warning signs of toxicity and will require attention from your doctor.* Check with your doctor immediately if you experience any of the following:
- confusion, severe drowsiness, slurred speech, severe weakness, unusual thoughts, shortness of breath, excitement, hyperactivity

Some side effects appear when you first start taking alprazolam and go away for most people. If the following side effects continue, contact your doctor.
- dizziness, lightheadedness, drowsiness, blurred vision, stomach problems

Drug Interactions
Alprazolam can adversely interact with the following frequently prescribed medications:
- cimetidine (Tagamet)—can cause high alprazolam levels
- disulfiram (Antabuse)—can cause high alprazolam levels
- birth control pills—can cause high alprazolam levels
- alcohol and other drugs that depress certain functions of the nervous system, when combined with alprazolam, cause extreme drowsiness and slowed reaction times. Examples of these medicines are antihistamines, narcotics, and barbiturates.
- levodopa—decreased effectiveness of levodopa

MEDICAL CONSIDERATIONS
If you have any of the following medical conditions, make sure your doctor is aware of it.

- liver disease or alcoholism—alprazolam levels may be higher than expected
- kidney disease—alprazolam levels may be higher than expected
- drug or alcohol dependence—dependence on alprazolam may occur
- seizure disorder—stopping alprazolam abruptly may cause seizures
- chronic lung disease—alprazolam may make breathing more difficult

---

Drug Name: AMITRIPTYLINE   (a-mee-TRIP-ti-leen)

Drug Category: Antidepressant, tricyclic
Requires prescription

Commonly Used Brand-Name Products
Tablets
Elavil (and generic) 10 mg, 25 mg, 50 mg, 75 mg, 100 mg, 150 mg
Injection
Elavil (and generic) 10 mg/ml

GENERAL INFORMATION
Highly effective in treating major depression and the depressed phase of bipolar disorder. Due to its sedative effects, it is sometimes given in low doses for insomnia. It is also used to treat certain chronic pain disorders, such as migraine headache and diabetic neuropathy.

Before Taking this Medication
Talk to your doctor about the benefits and risks associated with amitriptyline. Make sure you understand how to take it safely and effectively. Make sure your doctor has the following information in detail:

- any allergic or bad reactions you have had to amitriptyline or any other medication
- all prescription and over-the-counter medicines you are taking
- your complete medical history
- if you are pregnant, could be pregnant, or are planning a pregnancy in the near future, amitriptyline has not been shown to be absolutely safe

- if you are breast-feeding, amitriptyline can pass into breast milk and affect the baby

DOSAGE

The starting dose of amitriptyline will be low and gradually be increased. Sometimes blood levels are tested to ensure the dose you are taking is in the safe and effective range.

Adults:

Depression: Starting dose 25–50 mg at bedtime. Increased to 75–300 mg at bedtime over 2 to 3 weeks.

Insomnia: 25–100 mg at bedtime.

Chronic pain syndromes: 25–100 mg daily.

Adolescents: Adolescents may be more susceptible to heart-related side effects. Blood levels and heart function should be monitored.

Children under 12: Safe use and dosages in this age group have not been established. Children are more susceptible to serious heart-related side effects. Blood levels and heart function should be monitored.

Older adults are more susceptible to side effects and generally require lower dosages.

DIRECTIONS FOR PROPER USE

- *Take exactly as prescribed. Do not take more or less than prescribed. Accidental or intended overdoses of amitriptyline are potentially fatal.*
- If you miss a bedtime dose, do not take it the next morning. It may make you drowsy. Do not double doses.
- It may take several weeks before you feel the full benefits.
- Do not abruptly stop taking amitriptyline unless instructed to do so by your doctor. Gradually reducing the dose can help prevent mood changes, headache, or diarrhea.

PRECAUTIONS

Alcohol can cause changes in mood and may interfere with amitriptyline's effectiveness. *Alcohol should be avoided while taking amitriptyline.*

Side Effects

Not all side effects will occur. Many side effects will diminish with time. *However, some side effects may require attention from your doctor.* Check with your doctor immediately if you experience any of the following:

- seizure, changes in blood pressure, irregular heart rate, shortness of breath, problems with urination, (difficult or painful urination; unable to urinate), confusion, extreme sedation, excitation or mania, increased skin sensitivity to the sunlight, extreme constipation, yellow skin or eyes

Some side effects appear when you first start taking amitriptyline and go away for most people. If the following side effects continue, contact your doctor.

- dizziness, blurred vision, dry mouth, mild to moderate constipation, increased appetite, weight gain, breast enlargement (men or women), discharge from the breast, sexual problems, hand tremors, persistent sore throat

Drug Interactions
Amitriptyline can adversely interact with the following frequently prescribed medications:

- cimetidine (Tagamet)—can cause high amitriptyline levels
- SSRI antidepressants—can cause high amitriptyline levels
- MAOI antidepressants—severe reaction causing dangerously high blood pressure, high body temperature, seizures, or death
- clonidine—if clonidine is being taken for high blood pressure, amitriptyline may cause clonidine to work less well
- antipsychotics—may increase certain neurologic side effects
- thyroid hormones—increased effects of both, especially excitation and changes in heart rate or rhythm
- drugs used during surgery—can cause increased blood pressure. Make sure your doctors are aware of upcoming planned surgeries

MEDICAL CONSIDERATIONS
If you have any of the following medical conditions, make sure your doctor is aware of it.

- liver disease or alcoholism—amitriptyline levels may be higher than expected
- kidney disease—amitriptyline levels may be higher than expected
- glaucoma—amitriptyline can increase pressure inside the eye
- heart problems—some heart problems can be worsened by amitriptyline. It should not be taken by someone who has had a recent heart attack
- urinary retention, prostate enlargement—urination may become more difficult
- seizure disorder—amitriptyline can lower seizure threshold

- diabetes mellitus (sugar diabetes)—blood sugar levels may be affected
- thyroid disorders—amitriptyline may cause increased heart rate

---

Drug Name: AMOXAPINE   (a-MOX-a-peen)

Drug Category: Antidepressant, tricyclic
Requires prescription

Commonly Used Brand-Name Products
Tablets Asendin (and generic) 25 mg, 50 mg, 100 mg, 150 mg

GENERAL INFORMATION
Highly effective in treating major depression and the depressed phase of bipolar disorder.

Before Taking this Medication
Talk to your doctor about the benefits and risks associated with amoxapine. Make sure you understand how to take it safely and effectively. Make sure your doctor has the following information in detail:

- any allergic or bad reactions you have had to amoxapine or any other medication
- all prescription and over-the-counter medicines you are taking
- your complete medical history
- if you are pregnant, could be pregnant, or are planning a pregnancy in the near future, amoxapine has not been shown to be absolutely safe
- if you are breast-feeding, amoxapine can pass into breast milk and affect the baby

DOSAGE
The starting dose of amoxapine will be low and gradually be increased.

Adults: Starting dose 50 mg at bedtime. Increased to 150–300 mg at bedtime over 2 to 3 weeks.

Adolescents over 16: Adolescents may be more susceptible to heart-related side effects. Heart function should be monitored.

Children up to 16: Safe use and dosages in this age group have not been established.

<u>Older adults</u> are more susceptible to side effects and generally will require lower dosages.

DIRECTIONS FOR PROPER USE

- *Take exactly as prescribed. Do not take more or less than prescribed. Accidental or intended overdoses of amoxapine are potentially fatal.*
- If you miss a bedtime dose, do not take it the next morning. It may make you drowsy. Do not double doses.
- It may take several weeks before you feel the full benefits.
- Do not abruptly stop taking amoxapine unless instructed to do so by your doctor. Gradually reducing the dose can help prevent mood changes, headache, or diarrhea.

PRECAUTIONS

Alcohol can cause changes in mood and may interfere with amoxapine's effectiveness. *Alcohol should be avoided while taking amoxapine.*

Side Effects

Not all side effects will occur. Many side effects will diminish with time. *However, some side effects may require attention from your doctor.* Check with your doctor immediately if you experience any of the following:

- seizure, changes in blood pressure, irregular heart rate, shortness of breath, problems with urination, (difficult or painful urination; unable to urinate), confusion, extreme sedation, excitation or mania, severe skin sensitivity to sunlight (burning or blistering), extreme constipation, yellow skin or eyes
- lip puckering or lip smacking, uncontrolled movements of the tongue, uncontrolled movements of the hands, arms or legs, difficulty walking, rigid or stiff muscles, fever

Some side effects appear when you first start taking amoxapine and go away for most people. If the following side effects continue, contact your doctor.

- dizziness, blurred vision, dry mouth, mild to moderate constipation, increased appetite, weight gain, breast enlargement (men or women), discharge from the breast, sexual problems, hand tremor, persistent sore throat

Drug Interactions

Amoxapine can adversely interact with the following frequently prescribed medications:

- cimetidine (Tagamet)—can cause high amoxapine levels
- SSRI antidepressants—can cause high amoxapine levels
- MAOI antidepressants—severe reaction causing dangerously high blood pressure, high body temperature, seizures, or death
- clonidine—if clonidine is being taken for high blood pressure, amoxapine may cause it to work less well
- antipsychotics—may increase certain neurologic side effects
- thyroid hormones—increased effects of both, especially excitation and changes in heart rate or rhythm
- drugs used during surgery—can cause increased blood pressure. Make sure your doctors are aware of upcoming planned surgeries

MEDICAL CONSIDERATIONS
If you have any of the following medical conditions, make sure your doctor is aware of it.

- liver disease or alcoholism—amoxapine levels may be higher than expected
- kidney disease—amoxapine levels may be higher than expected
- glaucoma—amoxapine can increase pressure inside the eye
- heart problems—some heart problems can be worsened by amoxapine. It should not be taken by someone who has had a recent heart attack
- urinary retention, prostate enlargement—urination may become more difficult
- seizure disorder—amoxapine can lower seizure threshold
- diabetes mellitus (sugar diabetes)—blood sugar levels may be affected
- thyroid disorders—amoxapine may cause increased heart rate

Drug Name: AMPHETAMINE   (am-FET-a-meen)

Drug Category: Stimulant
Controlled substance, high potential for abuse, requires special prescription (triplicate, nonrefillable)

Commonly Used Brand-Name Products
Amphetamine—**tablets** 5 mg and 10 mg
Dextroamphetamine—Dexedrine (and generic) **tablets** 5 mg and 10 mg
Dexedrine (and generic) **long-acting capsules** 5 mg, 10 mg, and 15 mg
Methamphetamine—Desoxyn 5 mg **tablets** and **long-acting tablets** 5 mg, 10 mg, and 15 mg
Amphetamine mixture—Adderall, **tablets** 10 mg, and 20 mg

GENERAL INFORMATION
Highly effective in treating Attention Deficit Disorder and narcolepsy (uncontrolled need for sleep or suddenly falling into deep sleep). Amphetamines can sometimes be used to treat major depression.

Before Taking this Medication
Talk to your doctor about the benefits and risks associated with amphetamines. Make sure you understand how to take them safely and effectively. Make sure your doctor has the following information in detail:

- any allergic or bad reactions you have had to amphetamines or any other medication
- all prescription and over-the-counter medicines you are taking
- your complete medical history
- if you are pregnant, could be pregnant, or are planning a pregnancy in the near future, amphetamines have not been shown to be absolutely safe
- if you are breast-feeding, amphetamines can pass into breast milk and affect the baby

DOSAGE
The starting dose of amphetamines will be low and gradually be increased.

Adults and children over 6: 5 mg to 20 mg 2 to 3 times daily.

Older adults are more susceptible to side effects and will generally require lower dosages.

DIRECTIONS FOR PROPER USE
- *Take exactly as prescribed. Do not take more or less than prescribed. Accidental or intended overdoses of amphetamines are very serious.*

- If you miss a dose of the regular tablets, take it as soon as possible, unless it is within 3 hours of your next scheduled dose, then skip the missed dose and resume with your next scheduled dose. If you miss a dose of the long-acting tablets, skip the dose and resume with your next scheduled dose. Do not double doses.
- To prevent trouble sleeping do not take the last dose later than 6 pm for regular tablets and 3 pm for long-acting tablets, unless otherwise directed by your doctor.
- If you are taking the long-acting form, the tablets or capsules should be swallowed whole. Do not crush, break, or chew them.
- Do not abruptly stop taking amphetamines unless instructed to do so by your doctor.

PRECAUTIONS

Amphetamines can mask some of the effects of alcohol. Routine alcohol use, or alcohol withdrawal, can increase the chance of seizures, as can amphetamines. *Alcohol should be avoided while taking amphetamines.*

Side Effects

Not all side effects will occur. Many side effects will diminish with time. *However, some side effects may require attention from your doctor.* Check with your doctor immediately if you experience any of the following:

- seizure, increased blood pressure, fast or irregular heart rate, shortness of breath, confusion, excitation or mania, severe headache, muscle twitching, unusual behavior, depressed mood, rash or itching

Some side effects appear when you first start taking amphetamines and go away for most people. If the following side effects continue, contact your doctor.

- dizziness, nervousness, blurred vision, difficulty sleeping, decreased appetite, weight loss

Drug Interactions

Amphetamines can adversely interact with the following frequently prescribed medications:

- MAOI antidepressants—severe reaction causing dangerously high blood pressure, high body temperature, seizures, or death
- other stimulant medicines—decongestants, diet pills, some asthma medications, caffeine

- thyroid medications—the effects of thyroid medicines may be increased
- tricyclic antidepressants—increased blood pressure, irregular heart rate, or very high fever may result
- beta blockers—high blood pressure or decreased heart rate may result
- meperidine—extremely low blood pressure, slowed breathing, or very high fever may result

MEDICAL CONSIDERATIONS
If you have any of the following medical conditions, make sure your doctor is aware of it.

- liver disease or alcoholism—amphetamines levels may be higher than expected
- seizure disorder—amphetamines may increase the chance of seizures
- kidney disease—amphetamine levels may be higher than expected
- alcohol or drug abuse—dependence on amphetamines may result
- heart problems—some heart problems can be worsened by amphetamines
- glaucoma—may raise intraocular pressure
- high blood pressure—amphetamines may increase blood pressure
- Tourette's syndrome—amphetamines may worsen tics
- hyperthyroidism—thyroid hormone levels may increase

Drug Category: ANTICHOLINERGICS/ANTIDYSKINETICS
Requires prescription

Commonly Used Brand-Name Products	
Benztropine (Cogentin) Trihexyphenidyl (Artane)	Amantadine (Symmetrel)

GENERAL INFORMATION
Anticholinergics are used to treat side effects caused by other medicines, such as hand tremor or severe restlessness. They are also used to treat Parkinson's disease.

Before Taking this Medication

Talk to your doctor about the benefits and risks associated with anticholinergic medicine. Your doctor will need to know your complete medical history before prescribing an anticholinergic. Your doctor or pharmacist will need to be aware of all medicines that you take to avoid any drug interactions with an anticholinergic. Make sure you understand how to take an anticholinergic. Do not take more or less than prescribed. Do not suddenly stop taking an anticholinergic, unless directed by your doctor.

PRECAUTIONS

Alcohol should be avoided while taking anticholinergics.

Side Effects

Not all side effects will occur. Many side effects will diminish with time. *However, some side effects may be warning signs of toxicity and will require attention from your doctor.* Check with your doctor immediately if you experience any of the following:

- confusion, extreme dizziness or light-headedness, fast heart rate, eye pain, difficulty urinating, difficulty swallowing, rash or itching, unusual excitement, extreme restlessness

Some side effects appear when you first start taking anticholinergics and go away for most people. If the following side effects continue, contact your doctor.

- blurred vision, severe fatigue, dry mouth, flushing of the skin, constipation

---

Drug Category: ANTIHISTAMINES

Some require prescription. Some are over-the-counter.

Commonly Used Brand-Name Products	
Diphenhydramine (Benadryl)	Hydroxyzine (Vistaril, Atarax)

GENERAL INFORMATION

Antihistamines can help some people treat anxiety symptoms or insomnia. They are also used to treat allergic conditions.

Before Taking this Medication

Talk to your doctor about the benefits and risks associated with antihistamines. Your doctor will need to know your complete medical history before prescribing an antihistamine. Your doctor or pharmacist will need to be aware of all medicines that you take to avoid any drug interactions with an antihistamine. Make sure you understand how to take an antihistamine. Do not take more or less than prescribed. Do not suddenly stop taking an antihistamine, unless directed by your doctor.

PRECAUTIONS
Alcohol should be avoided while taking antihistamines.

Side Effects
Not all side effects will occur. Many side effects will diminish with time. *However, some side effects may be warning signs of toxicity and will require attention from your doctor.* Check with your doctor immediately if you experience any of the following:

- confusion, extreme dizziness or light-headedness, difficulty urinating, rash or itching, unusual excitement, extreme restlessness, fast heart rate

Some side effects appear when you first start taking antihistamines and go away for most people. If the following side effects continue, contact your doctor.

- blurred vision, severe fatigue, dry mouth, flushing of the skin, constipation

---

Drug Category: BETA BLOCKERS
Requires prescription

Commonly Used Brand-Name Products	
Atenolol (Tenormin) Metoprolol (Lopressor)	Nadolol (Corgard) Pindolol (Visken) Propranolol (Inderal)

GENERAL INFORMATION
Beta blockers are used to help relieve certain symptoms of panic disorder, such as increased heart rate. They also can be used to treat side effects resulting from other medicines, such as hand tremor, severe restlessness, and sometimes are used to relieve severe anxiety symptoms associated with stressful situations like public speaking. Beta blockers are primarily used to treat a variety of conditions, such as high blood pressure, irregular heart rate,

and heart disease. Your doctor will need to know your complete medical history before prescribing a beta blocker.

Before Taking this Medication

Talk to your doctor about the benefits and risks associated with beta blockers. Your doctor or pharmacist will need to be aware of all medicines that you take to avoid any drug interactions with a beta blocker. Make sure you understand how to take a beta blocker. Do not take more or less than prescribed. Do not suddenly stop taking a beta blocker, unless directed by your doctor.

PRECAUTIONS

Alcohol should be avoided while taking beta blockers.

Side Effects

Not all side effects will occur. Many side effects will diminish with time. *However, some side effects may be warning signs of toxicity and will require attention from your doctor.* Check with your doctor immediately if you experience any of the following:

- difficulty breathing, depressed mood, slow heart rate, irregular heart rate, chest pain, dizziness, light-headedness, swelling of the feet or ankles, confusion, extreme fatigue, sweating

Some side effects appear when you first start taking beta blockers and go away for most people. If the following side effects continue, contact your doctor.

- mild fatigue, dizziness, sexual problems

Drug Name: BUPROPION   (bewe-PRO-pe-on)

Drug Category: Antidepressant, atypical
Requires prescription

Commonly Used Brand-Name Products
Tablets
Wellbutrin 75 mg, 100 mg
Tablets, sustained released
Wellbutrin SR 100 mg, 150 mg

GENERAL INFORMATION

Highly effective in treating major depression, and the depressed phase of bipolar disorder. Effective in treating Attention Deficit Disorder.

Before Taking this Medication

Talk to your doctor about the benefits and risks associated with bupropion. Make sure you understand how to take it safely and effectively. Make sure your doctor has the following information in detail:

- any allergic or bad reactions you have had to bupropion or any other medication
- all prescription and over-the-counter medicines you are taking
- your complete medical history
- if you are pregnant, could be pregnant, or are planning a pregnancy in the near future, bupropion has not been shown to be absolutely safe
- if you are breast-feeding, bupropion can pass into breast milk and affect the baby

DOSAGE

The starting dose of bupropion will be low and gradually be increased.

<u>Adults:</u> Regular tablets: 75–150 mg 2 to 3 times daily.

Sustained release tablets: 100–150 mg 1 or 2 times daily.

<u>Older adults</u> are more susceptible to side effects and generally require lower dosages.

<u>Children and adolescents under 18:</u> Safe use and dosages have not been established in this age group.

DIRECTIONS FOR PROPER USE

- *Take exactly as prescribed. Do not take more or less than prescribed. Accidental or intended overdoses of bupropion are potentially fatal. Bupropion is associated with a higher occurrence of seizures than other antidepressants. Taking bupropion exactly as directed can reduce the risk of seizures. Bupropion, sustained release, does not have a higher incidence of seizures than other antidepressants.*
- Take with food or milk to lessen stomach upset.
- Check with your doctor about what to do if you miss a dose. Do not double doses.
- Doses of bupropion tablets should always be 4 to 6 hours apart. Doses of sustained release bupropion should be 8 hours apart.

- It may take several weeks before you feel the full benefits.
- Do not abruptly stop taking bupropion unless instructed to do so by your doctor. Gradually reducing the dose can help prevent mood changes, headache, or diarrhea.

PRECAUTIONS

Alcohol can cause changes in mood and may interfere with bupropion's effectiveness. Routine alcohol use, or alcohol withdrawal, can increase the chances of seizures. *Alcohol should be avoided while taking bupropion.*

Side Effects

Not all side effects will occur. Many side effects will diminish with time. *However, some side effects may require attention from your doctor.* Check with your doctor immediately if you experience any of the following:

- seizure, changes in blood pressure, irregular heart rate, shortness of breath, problems with urination, (difficult or painful urination; unable to urinate), confusion, extreme sedation, excitation or mania, extreme constipation, yellow skin or eyes, significant weight loss, severe headache

Some side effects appear when you first start taking bupropion and go away for most people. If the following side effects continue, contact your doctor.

- dizziness, blurred vision, dry mouth, mild to moderate constipation, increased appetite, weight gain, tremor of the hands

Drug Interactions

Bupropion can adversely interact with the following frequently prescribed medications:

- SSRI antidepressants—can cause high bupropion levels
- MAOI antidepressants—severe reaction causing dangerously high blood pressure, high body temperature, seizures, or death
- clonidine—if clonidine is being taken for high blood pressure, bupropion may cause it to work less well
- antipsychotics—may increase certain neurologic side effects
- drugs used during surgery—can cause increased blood pressure. Make sure your doctors are aware of upcoming planned surgeries

MEDICAL CONSIDERATIONS

If you have any of the following medical conditions, make sure your doctor is aware of it.

- liver disease or alcoholism—bupropion levels may be higher than expected
- seizure disorder—bupropion may increase the chance of seizures
- kidney disease—bupropion levels may be higher than expected
- heart problems—some heart problems can be worsened by bupropion. It should not be taken by someone who has had a recent heart attack
- urinary retention, prostate enlargement—urination may become more difficult
- bulimia or anorexia—there is an increased risk of seizure

Drug Name: BUSPIRONE   (byou-SPI-rone)

Drug Category: Antianxiety medicine
Requires prescription

Commonly Used Brand-Name Products
Tablets BuSpar 5 mg and 10 mg

GENERAL INFORMATION
Effective in treating anxiety and nervousness.

Before Taking this Medication
Talk to your doctor about the benefits and risks associated with buspirone. Make sure you understand how to take it safely and effectively. You and your family members should be very familiar with the side effects and signs of having too much in your system. Make sure your doctor has the following information in detail:

- any allergic or bad reactions you have had to buspirone or any other medication
- all prescription and over-the-counter medicines you are taking
- your complete medical history
- if you are pregnant, could be pregnant, or are planning a pregnancy in the near future, buspirone should not be taken
- if you are breast-feeding, buspirone can pass into breast milk and affect the baby

DOSAGE
<u>Adults:</u> 5 mg to 10 mg 2 to 3 times a day.

<u>Older adults</u> are more susceptible to side effects and generally require lower dosages.

<u>Children under 18:</u> Safe use has not been established in this age group.

DIRECTIONS FOR PROPER USE

- *Take exactly as prescribed. Do not take more or less than prescribed. Buspirone levels that are too high can cause serious toxicity.*
- Several weeks may elapse before you begin to feel the full benefit of buspirone.
- If you take buspirone regularly for an extended period of time, do not stop taking it unless told to do so by your doctor. It may be necessary to gradually reduce the dose before stopping completely.
- If you miss a dose, take it as soon as possible. However, if the missed dose is within 4 hours of your next dose, skip the missed dose and resume with your next scheduled dose.

PRECAUTIONS

Alcohol should be avoided while taking buspirone.

Side Effects

Not all side effects will occur. Many side effects will diminish with time. *However, some side effects may be warning signs of toxicity and will require attention from your doctor.* Check with your doctor immediately if you experience any of the following:

- confusion, depressed mood, severe drowsiness, slurred speech, severe weakness, unusual thoughts, shortness of breath, excitement, extreme muscle pain or stiffness, severe nausea, vomiting

Some side effects appear when you first start taking buspirone and go away for most people. If the following side effects continue, contact your doctor.

- dizziness, light-headedness, drowsiness, blurred vision, stomach problems, sexual problems

Drug Interactions

Buspirone can adversely interact with the following frequently prescribed medications:

- monoamine oxidase inhibitors—a severe reaction causing dangerously high blood pressure, high body temperature, seizures, or death, is possible

- alcohol and other drugs that depress certain functions of the nervous system, when combined with buspirone, can cause extreme drowsiness and slowed reaction times. Examples of these medicines are antihistamines, narcotics, and barbiturates.

MEDICAL CONSIDERATIONS
If you have any of the following medical conditions, make sure your doctor is aware of it.

- liver disease or alcoholism—buspirone levels may be higher than expected
- kidney disease—buspirone levels may be higher than expected

---

Drug Name: CARBAMAZEPINE   (car-ba-MAZ-e-peen)

Drug Category: Mood stabilizer
Requires prescription

Commonly Used Brand-Name Products
Tablets
Tegretol 100 mg chewable tablets (and generic)
Tegretol 200 mg tablets (and generic)
Extended release tablets
Tegretol XR 100 mg, 200 mg and 400 mg
Tegretol suspension 100 mg/teaspoonful

GENERAL INFORMATION
Very effective for treating bipolar disorder (manic-depressive disorder), especially hard to treat cases, such as rapid cycling. Also reduces the number and severity of subsequent episodes of both mania and depression. Can be used alone, or in combination with other mood stabilizers. It is also used to treat schizoaffective disorder, usually in combination with other medications called antipsychotics. There is some evidence that carbamazepine can help people who have significant problems with impulse control, by reducing anger, temper outbursts, or aggressive behaviors.

Before Taking this Medication
Talk to your doctor about the benefits and risks associated with carbamazepine. Make sure you understand how to take it safely and effectively. You and your family members should be very familiar with the side effects and signs of having too much in your

system. Make sure your doctor has the following information in detail:

- any allergic or bad reactions you have had to carbamazepine or any other medication
- all prescription and over-the-counter medicines you are taking
- your complete medical history
- if you are pregnant, could be pregnant, or are planning a pregnancy in the near future, carbamazepine should be avoided
- if you are breast-feeding, carbamazepine can pass into breast milk and affect the baby

DOSAGE

When you first start taking carbamazepine, your dose will be adjusted based on your response and blood levels.

Adults and adolescents: 600–1600 mg per day, divided in 2 to 4 doses daily.

Older adults are more susceptible to side effects and generally require lower dosages.

Children 6 to 12: dosages in this age group are lower than those for adults.

Children up to 6: dosage is based on body weight.

DIRECTIONS FOR PROPER USE

- *Take exactly as prescribed. Do not take more or less than prescribed. Carbamazepine levels that are too high can cause serious toxicity.*
- Take carbamazepine with meals or a snack. This will reduce stomach upset or diarrhea.
- If you take the liquid form, it should be shaken well to disperse all the medication evenly.
- If you miss a dose of the regular tablet or liquid form, take it as soon as possible. However, if it is very close to the time for the next dose, skip the missed dose and resume with the next scheduled dose. Do not double doses.
- If you are taking a long-acting form:
  - Swallow the tablet whole. Do not crush, split, or chew it.
  - If you miss a dose, take it as soon as possible. However, if the missed dose is within 6 hours of your next dose, skip the missed dose and resume with the next scheduled dose.
  - Long-acting tablets are not interchangeable with regular carbamazepine tablets, capsules, or liquid forms.
- It may take several weeks before you feel the full benefits.

- Laboratory tests are necessary to determine if the amount of carbamazepine in your bloodstream is in the correct range.

PRECAUTIONS

Alcohol can cause changes in mood and may interfere with carbamazepine's effectiveness. Routine alcohol use, or alcohol withdrawal, can increase the chances of seizures. *Alcohol should be avoided while taking carbamazepine.*

Side Effects

Not all side effects will occur. Many side effects will diminish with time. *However, some side effects may be warning signs of toxicity and will require attention from your doctor.* Check with your doctor immediately if you experience any of the following:

- unusual bleeding or bruising, black stools, blood in the urine, difficulty urinating, confusion, significant drowsiness, irregular heart beat, difficulty breathing, swelling of the feet or hands, yellow eyes or skin, fever

Check with your doctor as soon as possible for the following side effects:

- back-and-forth movement of the eyes, blurred or double vision, skin rash or hives, severe diarrhea

Some side effects appear when you first start taking carbamazepine and go away for most people. If the following side effects continue, contact your doctor.

- mild hand tremor, mild nausea, mild dizziness, diarrhea or constipation, increased sensitivity of skin to sunlight, dry mouth

Drug Interactions

Carbamazepine can adversely interact with the following frequently prescribed medications:

- anticoagulants (blood thinners)—the effect of the anticoagulant can be decreased
- certain medications for high blood pressure such as calcium channel blockers—can cause increased carbamazepine levels
- cimetidine (Tagamet)—carbamazepine levels can be increased
- erythromycin and similar antibiotics—can cause increased carbamazepine levels
- propoxyphene (Darvon)—carbamazepine levels can be increased
- birth control pills—carbamazepine may cause birth control pills to work less well

- tricyclic antidepressants—increased sedation, change in blood levels of carbamazepine or the antidepressant

MEDICAL CONSIDERATIONS

If you have any of the following medical conditions, make sure your doctor is aware of it.

- liver disease or alcoholism—carbamazepine levels may be higher than expected
- kidney disease—carbamazepine levels may be higher than expected
- anemia or other blood problems—these conditions can be worsened by carbamazepine
- heart problems—some heart problems can be worsened by carbamazepine, usually in the elderly
- problems with urination—carbamazepine may worsen this condition
- glaucoma—carbamazepine may worsen this condition
- diabetes mellitus (sugar diabetes)—urine sugar levels may increase

---

Drug Name: CHLORDIAZEPOXIDE   (klor-dye-AZ-ep-ox-ide)

Drug Category: Antianxiety medicine

Requires prescription, controlled substance, moderate potential for abuse

Commonly Used Brand-Name Products
Capsules Librium (and generic) 5 mg, 10 mg, and 25 mg **Tablets** Libritabs 5 mg, 10 mg, and 25 mg **Injection** 100 mg/2ml

GENERAL INFORMATION

Highly effective in treating anxiety and nervousness and is also used to treat symptoms of alcohol withdrawal.

Before Taking this Medication

Talk to your doctor about the benefits and risks associated with chlordiazepoxide. Make sure you understand how to take it safely and effectively. You and your family members should be very familiar with the side effects and signs of having too much in your system. Make sure your doctor has the following information in detail:

- any allergic or bad reactions you have had to chlordiazepoxide or any other medication
- all prescription and over-the-counter medicines you are taking
- your complete medical history
- if you are pregnant, could be pregnant, or are planning a pregnancy in the near future, chlordiazepoxide should not be taken.
- if you are breast-feeding, chlordiazepoxide can pass into breast milk and affect the baby

DOSAGE
<u>Adults:</u> 5 to 25 mg 2 to 4 times a day.
<u>Older adults</u> are more susceptible to side effects and generally require lower dosages.
<u>Children over 6:</u> When used in children, dosage is based on body weight.
<u>Children under 6:</u> Dosages in this age group have not been established.

DIRECTIONS FOR PROPER USE
- *Take exactly as prescribed. Do not take more or less than prescribed. Chlordiazepoxide levels that are too high can cause serious toxicity.*
- Take with food if stomach upset occurs.
- If you take chlordiazepoxide regularly for an extended period of time, do not stop taking it unless told to do so by your doctor. It may be necessary to gradually reduce the dose before stopping completely.
- If you miss a dose, take it as soon as possible. However, if the missed dose is within 6 hours of your next dose, skip the missed dose and resume with your next scheduled dose.

PRECAUTIONS
Alcohol should be avoided while taking chlordiazepoxide.

Side Effects
Not all side effects will occur. Many side effects will diminish with time. *However, some side effects may be warning signs of toxicity and will require attention from your doctor.* Check with your doctor immediately if you experience any of the following:

- confusion, severe drowsiness, slurred speech, severe weakness, unusual thoughts, shortness of breath, excitement, hyperactivity

Some side effects appear when you first start taking chlordiazepoxide and go away for most people. If the following side effects continue, contact your doctor.

- dizziness, light-headedness, drowsiness, blurred vision, stomach problems

Drug Interactions

Chlordiazepoxide can adversely interact with the following frequently prescribed medications:

- cimetidine (Tagamet)—can cause high chlordiazepoxide levels
- disulfiram (Antabuse)—can cause high chlordiazepoxide levels
- birth control pills—can cause high chlordiazepoxide levels
- alcohol and other drugs that depress certain functions of the nervous system, when combined with chlordiazepoxide, can cause extreme drowsiness and slowed reaction times. Examples of these medicines are antihistamines, narcotics, and barbiturates.
- levodopa—decreased effectiveness of levodopa

MEDICAL CONSIDERATIONS

If you have any of the following medical conditions, make sure your doctor is aware of it.

- liver disease or alcoholism—chlordiazepoxide levels may be higher than expected
- kidney disease—chlordiazepoxide levels may be higher than expected
- drug dependence or alcohol dependence—dependence on chlordiazepoxide may occur
- seizure disorder—stopping chlordiazepoxide abruptly may cause seizures
- chronic lung disease—chlordiazepoxide may make breathing more difficult

---

Drug Name: CHLORPROMAZINE   (klor-PRO-ma-zeen)

Drug Category: Neuroleptic; Antipsychotic
Requires prescription

Commonly Used Brand-Name Products	
Tablets Thorazine (and generic) 10 mg, 25 mg, 50 mg, 100 mg, 200 mg **Long-acting capsules** Thorazine spansule 30 mg, 75 mg, 150 mg, 200 mg, 300 mg **Injection** Thorazine (and generic) 25 mg/ml	**Liquids,** Thorazine (and generic) Syrup, 10 mg/5ml Concentrate, 30 mg/ml and 100 mg/ml **Suppository** Thorazine 25 mg, 100 mg

GENERAL INFORMATION

Highly effective in treating psychotic symptoms, such as hallucinations and delusions. These symptoms occur in schizophrenia, schizoaffective disorder, bipolar disorder, or major depression with psychotic features. Chlorpromazine can be used for short-term management of aggressive, out-of-control behaviors or feelings of anger and rage. It is used to help with symptoms of anxiety and insomnia.

Before Taking this Medication

Talk to your doctor about the benefits and risks associated with chlorpromazine. Make sure you understand how to take it safely and effectively. You and your family members should be very familiar with its side effects. Make sure your doctor has the following information in detail:

- any allergic or bad reactions you have had to chlorpromazine or any other medication
- all prescription and over-the-counter medicines you are taking
- your complete medical history
- if you are pregnant, could be pregnant, or are planning a pregnancy in the near future, chlorpromazine has not been shown to be absolutely safe
- if you are breast-feeding, chlorpromazine can pass into breast milk and affect the baby

DOSAGE

Adults and adolescents:

Psychotic symptoms: 100–1600 mg daily. There is a wide effective dosage range.

Anxiety and insomnia: 25–100 mg, usually at bedtime, but for extreme anxiety can be given during waking hours.

Older adults are more susceptible to side effects and will generally require lower dosages.

Children under 12: Dosages in this age group have not been established.

DIRECTIONS FOR PROPER USE

- *Take exactly as prescribed. Do not take more or less than prescribed.*
- If you taking a liquid form, avoid contacting the skin with the medicine. Irritation can result by the medicine coming into contact with skin. Do not use the liquid form if the medicine becomes very discolored (dark yellow) or has a sediment at the bottom of the bottle.
- If you are taking the *concentrate* form, note that this is a strong form of chlorpromazine. Mix your dose in a half a glass of coffee, tea, milk, tomato or fruit juice before taking.
- If you miss a dose, take it as soon as possible. However, if the missed dose is within 4 hours of your next dose, skip the missed dose and resume with your next scheduled dose.
- If you are taking a long-acting form:
  - Swallow the capsule whole. Do not crush, open, or chew it.
  - If you miss a dose, take it as soon as possible. However, if the missed dose is within 6 hours of your next dose, skip the missed dose and resume with your next scheduled dose.
  - Long-acting capsules are not interchangeable with regular chlorpromazine tablets or liquid forms.
- It may take several weeks before you feel the full benefits.

PRECAUTIONS

Alcohol should be avoided while taking chlorpromazine.

Side Effects

Not all side effects will occur. Many side effects will diminish with time. *However, some side effects may be warning signs of toxicity and will require attention from your doctor.* Check with your doctor immediately if you experience any of the following:

- seizure, high fever, fast or irregular heartbeat, very low blood pressure, faintness, any abnormal movements of the mouth, tongue, neck, arms or legs, difficulty speaking or swallowing, imbalance or difficulty walking normally, severe muscle stiffness, discoloration of the skin or eyes, confusion, significant drowsiness, restlessness, difficulty urinating, sexual problems, vomiting, diarrhea, unusual bruising or bleeding, serious skin reaction to sunlight (burning or blistering), severe constipation, breast pain or enlargement

Some side effects appear when you first start taking chlorpromazine and go away for most people. If the following side effects continue, contact your doctor.

- dry mouth, mild to moderate constipation, dizziness, hand tremor, stuffy nose, weight gain

Drug Interactions
Chlorpromazine can adversely interact with the following frequently prescribed medications:

- lithium—increased neurologic side effects
- levodopa—decreased effectiveness of levodopa
- amphetamines—increased psychotic symptoms are possible
- anticonvulsants—decreased chlorpromazine levels
- tricyclic antidepressants—increased TCA levels

MEDICAL CONSIDERATIONS
If you have any of the following medical conditions, make sure your doctor is aware of it.

- kidney disease—chlorpromazine levels may be higher than expected
- liver disease—chlorpromazine levels may be higher than expected
- heart problems—some heart problems can be worsened by chlorpromazine
- seizure disorder—chlorpromazine can lower seizure threshold
- urinary retention, prostate enlargement—urination may be more difficult
- glaucoma—chlorpromazine can increase pressure inside the eye
- Parkinson's disease—some Parkinson's symptoms may be worsened
- breast cancer—may increase risk of cancer progression

Drug Name: CLOMIPRAMINE   (cloe-MIP-ra-meen)

Drug Category: Antidepressant, tricyclic
Requires prescription

Commonly Used Brand-Name Products
Capsules Anafranil 25 mg, 50 mg, 75 mg

GENERAL INFORMATION
Highly effective in treating obsessive compulsive disorder (OCD), also effective in treating major depression and the depressed phase of bipolar disorder.

Before Taking this Medication
Talk to your doctor about the benefits and risks associated with clomipramine. Make sure you understand how to take it safely and effectively. Make sure your doctor has the following information in detail:

- any allergic or bad reactions you have had to clomipramine or any other medication
- all prescription and over-the-counter medicines you are taking
- your complete medical history
- if you are pregnant, could be pregnant, or are planning a pregnancy in the near future, clomipramine has not been shown to be absolutely safe.
- if you are breast-feeding, clomipramine can pass into breast milk and affect the baby

DOSAGE
The starting dose of clomipramine will be low and gradually be increased. Sometimes blood levels are tested to ensure the dose you are taking is in the safe and effective range.

Adults:
> OCD, depression: Starting dose 25 mg at bedtime. Increased to 100–250 mg at bedtime over 2 to 3 weeks.

Children over 10 and adolescents (for OCD): Lower doses than for adults and based on body weight. Monitoring for heart-related side effects is recommended.

Children over 12 and adolescents (for depression): Lower doses than for adults and based on body weight.

Monitoring for heart-related side effects is recommended.

Older adults are more susceptible to side effects and generally require lower dosages.

DIRECTIONS FOR PROPER USE

- *Take exactly as prescribed. Do not take more or less than prescribed. Accidental or intended overdoses of clomipramine are potentially fatal.*
- Take with food or milk to reduce stomach upset.
- If you miss a bedtime dose, do not take it the next morning. It may make you drowsy. Do not double doses.
- It may take several weeks before you feel the full benefits.
- Do not abruptly stop taking clomipramine unless instructed to do so by your doctor. Gradually reducing the dose can help prevent mood changes, headache, or diarrhea.

PRECAUTIONS

Alcohol can cause changes in mood and may interfere with clomipramine's effectiveness. Routine alcohol use, or alcohol withdrawal, can increase the chances of seizures. *Alcohol should be avoided while taking clomipramine.*

Side Effects

Not all side effects will occur. Many side effects will diminish with time. *However, some side effects may require attention from your doctor.* Check with your doctor immediately if you experience any of the following:

- seizure, changes in blood pressure, irregular heart rate, shortness of breath, problems with urination, (difficult or painful urination; unable to urinate), confusion, extreme sedation, excitation or mania, severe skin sensitivity to sunlight (burning or blistering), extreme constipation, yellow skin or eyes

Some side effects appear when you first start taking clomipramine and go away for most people. If the following side effects continue, contact your doctor.

- dizziness, blurred vision, dry mouth, mild to moderate constipation, increased appetite, weight gain, breast enlargement (men or women), discharge from the breast, sexual problems, hand tremor, persistent sore throat

Drug Interactions

Clomipramine can adversely interact with the following frequently prescribed medications:

- cimetidine (Tagamet)—can cause high clomipramine levels
- SSRI antidepressants—can cause high clomipramine levels
- MAOI antidepressants—severe reaction causing dangerously high blood pressure, high body temperature, seizures, or death

- clonidine—if clonidine is being taken for high blood pressure, clomipramine may cause clonidine to work less well
- antipsychotics—may increase certain neurologic side effects
- thyroid hormones—increased effects of both, especially excitation and changes in heart rate or rhythm
- drugs used during surgery—can cause increased blood pressure. Make sure your doctors are aware of upcoming planned surgeries

MEDICAL CONSIDERATIONS

If you have any of the following medical conditions, make sure your doctor is aware of it.

- liver disease or alcoholism—clomipramine levels may be higher than expected
- kidney disease—clomipramine levels may be higher than expected
- glaucoma—clomipramine can increase pressure inside the eye
- heart problems—some heart problems can be worsened by clomipramine. It should not be taken by someone who has had a recent heart attack
- urinary retention, prostate enlargement—urination may become more difficult
- seizure disorder—clomipramine can lower seizure threshold
- diabetes mellitus (sugar diabetes)—blood sugar levels may be affected
- thyroid disorders—clomipramine may cause increased heart rate

---

Drug Name: CLONAZEPAM   (klon-AZ-e-pam)

Drug Category: Antianxiety medicine
Requires prescription, controlled substance, moderate potential for abuse

Commonly Used Brand-Name Products
Tablets
Klonopin (and generic) 0.5 mg, 1 mg, 2 mg

GENERAL INFORMATION

Highly effective in treating anxiety and nervousness. Also used to treat panic disorder and symptoms of alcohol withdrawal.

Before Taking this Medication

Talk to your doctor about the benefits and risks associated with clonazepam. Make sure you understand how to take clonazepam safely and effectively. You and your family members should be very familiar with the side effects and signs of having too much in your system. Make sure your doctor has the following information in detail:

- any allergic or bad reactions you have had to clonazepam or any other medication
- all prescription and over-the-counter medicines you are taking
- your complete medical history
- if you are pregnant, could be pregnant, or are planning a pregnancy in the near future, clonazepam should not be taken.
- if you are breast-feeding, clonazepam can pass into breast milk and affect the baby.

DOSAGE

<u>Adults:</u> 0.5 to 2 mg 2 to 3 times a day.

<u>Older adults</u> are more susceptible to side effects and generally require lower dosages.

<u>Children under 10:</u> When used in children, dosage is based on body weight.

DIRECTIONS FOR PROPER USE

- *Take exactly as prescribed. Do not take more or less than prescribed. Clonazepam levels that are too high can cause serious toxicity.*
- Take with food if stomach upset occurs.
- If you take clonazepam regularly for an extended period of time, do not stop taking it unless told to do so by your doctor. It may be necessary to gradually reduce the dose before stopping completely.
- If you miss a dose, take it as soon as possible. However, if the missed dose is within 6 hours of your next dose, skip the missed dose and resume with your next scheduled dose.

PRECAUTIONS

Alcohol should be avoided while taking clonazepam.

Side Effects

Not all side effects will occur. Many side effects will diminish with time. *However, some side effects may be warning signs of toxicity and will require attention from your doctor.* Check with your doctor immediately if you experience any of the following:

- confusion, severe drowsiness, slurred speech, severe weakness, unusual thoughts, shortness of breath, excitement, hyperactivity

Some side effects appear when you first start taking clonazepam and go away for most people. If the following side effects continue, contact your doctor.

- dizziness, light-headedness, drowsiness, blurred vision, stomach problems

Drug Interactions

Clonazepam can adversely interact with the following frequently prescribed medications:

- cimetidine (Tagamet)—can cause high clonazepam levels
- disulfiram (Antabuse)—can cause high clonazepam levels
- birth control pills—can cause high clonazepam levels
- alcohol and other drugs that depress certain functions of the nervous system, when combined with clonazepam, cause extreme drowsiness and slowed reaction times. Examples of these medicines are antihistamines, narcotics, and barbiturates.
- Levodopa—decreased effectiveness of levodopa

MEDICAL CONSIDERATIONS

If you have any of the following medical conditions, make sure your doctor is aware of it.

- liver disease or alcoholism—clonazepam levels may be higher than expected
- kidney disease—clonazepam levels may be higher than expected
- drug dependence or alcohol dependence—dependence on clonazepam may occur
- seizure disorder—stopping clonazepam abruptly may cause seizures
- chronic lung disease—clonazepam may make breathing more difficult

---

Drug Name: CLONIDINE   (Klon-A-deen)
Requires prescription

Commonly Used Brand-Name Products
Catapres (and generic), **tablets** and **skin patch**

GENERAL INFORMATION
Typically used to treat high blood pressure. It is sometimes used to treat aggression, hostility, or violent behaviors associated with a psychiatric or neurological disorder, and Attention Deficit Disorder.

Before Taking this Medication
Talk to your doctor about the benefits and risks associated with clonidine. Your doctor will need to know your complete medical history before prescribing clonidine. Your doctor or pharmacist will need to be aware of all medicines that you take to avoid any drug interactions with clonidine. Make sure you understand how to take it. Do not take more or less than prescribed. Do not abruptly stop taking clonidine, unless directed by your doctor.

PRECAUTIONS
Alcohol should be avoided while taking clonidine.

Side Effects
Not all side effects will occur. Many side effects will diminish with time. *However, some side effects may be warning signs of toxicity and will require attention from your doctor.* Check with your doctor immediately if you experience any of the following:

- difficulty breathing, slow heart rate, irregular heart rate, dizziness, light-headedness, swelling of the feet or ankles, confusion, extreme fatigue, red or itchy skin (especially wit the patch)

Some side effects appear when you first start taking clonidine and go away for most people. If the following side effects continue, contact your doctor.

- mild fatigue, dizziness, dry mouth, constipation

Drug Name: CLORAZEPATE   (klor-AZ-e-pate)

Drug Category: Antianxiety medicine
Requires prescription, controlled substance, moderate potential for abuse

Commonly Used Brand-Name Products
Tablets and Capsules Tranxene (and generic) 3.75 mg, 7.5 mg and 15 mg **Tablets, long-acting** Tranxene SD 11.25 mg, 22.5 mg

GENERAL INFORMATION

Highly effective in treating anxiety and nervousness. Also used to treat panic disorder and symptoms of alcohol withdrawal.

Before Taking this Medication

Talk to your doctor about the benefits and risks associated with clorazepate. Make sure you understand how to take it safely and effectively. You and your family members should be very familiar with the side effects and signs of having too much in your system. Make sure your doctor has the following information in detail:

- any allergic or bad reactions you have had to clorazepate or any other medication
- all prescription and over-the-counter medicines you are taking
- your complete medical history
- if you are pregnant, could be pregnant, or are planning a pregnancy in the near future, clorazepate should not be taken
- if you are breast-feeding, clorazepate can pass into breast milk and affect the baby

DOSAGE

<u>Adults:</u> 3.75–15 mg 2 to 4 times a day. The long-acting tablet form may be given once daily.

<u>Older adults</u> are more susceptible to side effects and generally require lower dosages.

<u>Children under 9:</u> Safe use has not been established in this age group.

DIRECTIONS FOR PROPER USE

- *Take exactly as prescribed. Do not take more or less than prescribed. Clorazepate levels that are too high can cause serious toxicity.*
- If you take clorazepate regularly for an extended period of time, do not stop taking it unless told to do so by your doctor. It may be necessary to gradually reduce the dose before stopping completely.
- If stomach upset occurs, clorazepate may be taken with food.

- If you miss a dose of the capsule or regular tablet form, take it as soon as possible. However, if the missed dose is within 6 hours of your next dose, skip the missed dose and resume with your next scheduled dose.
- If you are taking the long-acting tablet form and you miss a dose, take it as soon as possible within 1-2 hours of the missed dose. However, if it is more than 2 hours after the missed dose, skip the missed dose and resume with your next scheduled dose.

PRECAUTIONS
Alcohol should be avoided while taking clorazepate.

Side Effects
Not all side effects will occur. Many side effects will diminish with time. *However, some side effects may be warning signs of toxicity and will require attention from your doctor.* Check with your doctor immediately if you experience any of the following:

- confusion, severe drowsiness, slurred speech, severe weakness, unusual thoughts, shortness of breath, excitement, hyperactivity

Some side effects appear when you first start taking clorazepate and go away for most people. If the following side effects continue, contact your doctor.

- dizziness, light-headedness, drowsiness, blurred vision, stomach problems

Drug Interactions
Clorazepate can adversely interact with the following frequently prescribed medications:

- cimetidine (Tagamet)—can cause high clorazepate levels
- disulfiram (Antabuse)—can cause high clorazepate levels
- birth control pills—can cause high clorazepate levels
- alcohol and other drugs that depress certain functions of the nervous system, when combined with clorazepate, can cause extreme drowsiness and slowed reaction times. Examples of these medicines are antihistamines, narcotics, and barbiturates.
- levodopa—decreased effectiveness of levodopa

MEDICAL CONSIDERATIONS
If you have any of the following medical conditions, make sure your doctor is aware of it.

- liver disease or alcoholism—clorazepate levels may be higher than expected

- kidney disease—clorazepate levels may be higher than expected
- drug dependence or alcohol dependence—dependence on clorazepate may occur
- seizure disorder—stopping clorazepate abruptly may cause seizures
- chronic lung disease—clorazepate may make breathing more difficult

---

Drug Name: CLOZAPINE   (CLOZ-a-peen)

Drug Category: Neuroleptic; Antipsychotic
Requires prescription

Commonly Used Brand-Name Products
Tablets
Clozaril (and generic) 25 mg, 100 mg

GENERAL INFORMATION
Highly effective in treating schizophrenia, reducing psychotic symptoms, such as hallucinations and delusions. It is also especially helpful with symptoms such as lack of motivation, emotional blunting, and withdrawing from others.

Before Taking this Medication
Talk to your doctor about the benefits and risks associated with clozapine. Make sure you understand how to take it safely and effectively. You and your family members should be very familiar with the side effects. You and your family must be able to follow the special laboratory monitoring requirements necessary for safe use of clozapine. You will be able to receive only a 7-day supply of clozapine at a time and only if your blood tests show it is safe to continue taking. Make sure your doctor has the following information in detail:

- any allergic or bad reactions you have had to clozapine or any other medication
- all prescription and over-the-counter medicines you are taking
- your complete medical history
- if you are pregnant, could be pregnant, or are planning a pregnancy in the near future, clozapine has not been shown to be absolutely safe

- if you are breast-feeding, clozapine can pass into breast milk and affect the baby

DOSAGE

Adults and adolescents:

Psychotic symptoms: 300–900 mg daily.

Older adults are more susceptible to side effects and generally require lower dosages.

Children and adolescents under 16: Dosages in this age group have not been established.

DIRECTIONS FOR PROPER USE

- *Take exactly as prescribed. Do not take more or less than prescribed.*
- *Get laboratory tests done every week to check your white blood cell count. If you do not get these tests done, or if your white blood cell count drops too much, clozapine will have to be stopped.*
- If you miss a dose, take it as soon as possible. However, if the missed dose is within 4 hours of your next dose, skip the missed dose and resume with your next scheduled dose. Do not double doses.
- It may take several weeks before you feel the full benefits.

PRECAUTIONS

Alcohol should be avoided while taking clozapine.

Side Effects

Not all side effects will occur. Many side effects will diminish with time. *However, some side effects may be warning signs of toxicity and will require attention from your doctor.* Check with your doctor immediately if you experience any of the following:

- seizure, fast or irregular heartbeat, very low blood pressure, faintness, fever, sore throat, flu-like symptoms, any abnormal movements of the mouth, tongue, neck, arms or legs, difficulty speaking or swallowing, imbalance or difficulty walking normally, severe muscle stiffness, discoloration of the skin or eyes, confusion, significant drowsiness, restlessness, difficulty urinating, sexual problems, vomiting, diarrhea, unusual bruising or bleeding, serious skin reaction to sunlight (burning or blistering), severe constipation, breast pain or enlargement

Some side effects appear when you first start taking clozapine and go away for most people. If the following side effects continue, contact your doctor.

- increased salivation, dry mouth, nausea, mild to moderate constipation, dizziness, hand tremor, stuffy nose, weight gain

Drug Interactions
Clozapine can adversely interact with the following frequently prescribed medications:

- lithium—increased neurologic side effects
- levodopa—decreased effectiveness of levodopa
- amphetamines—increased psychotic symptoms are possible
- anticonvulsants—decreased clozapine levels
- tricyclic antidepressants—increased TCA levels
- cancer chemotherapy drugs—clozapine can interact to lower white blood cell count
- antiviral medicines (usually used to treat HIV)—clozapine can interact to lower white blood cell count

MEDICAL CONSIDERATIONS
If you have any of the following medical conditions, make sure your doctor is aware of it.

- kidney disease—clozapine levels may be higher than expected
- liver disease—clozapine levels may be higher than expected
- blood diseases—clozapine may make certain conditions worse
- heart problems—some heart problems can be worsened by clozapine
- seizure disorder—clozapine can lower seizure threshold
- urinary retention, prostate enlargement—urination may be more difficult
- glaucoma—clozapine can increase pressure inside the eye
- Parkinson's disease—some Parkinson's symptoms may be worsened
- breast cancer—may increase risk of cancer progression

Drug Name: DESIPRAMINE   (dess-IP-ra-meen)

Drug Category: Antidepressant, tricyclic
Requires prescription

Commonly Used Brand-Name Products
Tablets Norpramin (and generic) 10 mg, 25 mg, 50 mg, 100 mg, 150 mg

GENERAL INFORMATION

Highly effective in treating major depression, and the depressed phase of bipolar disorder. Very effective in treating panic disorder. Also used to treat attention deficit hyperactivity disorder, especially in adults, and certain chronic pain disorders, such as migraines and diabetic neuropathy.

Before Taking this Medication

Talk to your doctor about the benefits and risks associated with desipramine. Make sure you understand how to take it safely and effectively. Make sure your doctor has the following information in detail:

- any allergic or bad reactions you have had to desipramine or any other medication
- all prescription and over-the-counter medicines you are taking
- your complete medical history
- if you are pregnant, could be pregnant, or are planning a pregnancy in the near future, desipramine has not been shown to be absolutely safe
- if you are breast-feeding, desipramine can pass into breast milk and affect the baby

DOSAGE

The starting dose of desipramine will be low and gradually be increased. Sometimes blood levels can be tested to ensure the dose you are taking is in the safe and effective range.

<u>Adults:</u>
   <u>Depression, panic disorder, ADHD:</u> Starting dose 25–50 mg at bedtime. Increased to 75–300 mg at bedtime over 2 to 3 weeks.
   <u>Chronic pain syndromes:</u> 25–100 mg daily.

<u>Adolescents:</u> Adolescents may be more susceptible to heart-related side effects. Blood levels and heart function should be monitored.

<u>Children under 12:</u> Safe use and dosages for this age group have not been established. Children are more susceptible to serious heart-related side effects. Blood levels and heart function should be monitored.

<u>Older adults</u> are be more susceptible to side effects and generally require lower dosages.

DIRECTIONS FOR PROPER USE

- *Take exactly as prescribed. Do not take more or less than prescribed. Accidental or intended overdoses of desipramine are potentially fatal.*

- If you miss a bedtime dose, do not take it the next morning. It may make you drowsy. Do not double doses.
- It may take several weeks before you feel the full benefits.
- Laboratory tests may be done to determine if the amount of desipramine in your bloodstream is in the correct range.
- Do not abruptly stop taking desipramine unless instructed to do so by your doctor. Gradually reducing the dose can help prevent mood changes, headaches, or diarrhea.

PRECAUTIONS
Alcohol can cause changes in mood and may interfere with desipramine's effectiveness. *Alcohol should be avoided while taking desipramine.*

Side Effects
Not all side effects will occur. Many side effects will diminish with time. *However, some side effects may be warning signs of toxicity and will require attention from your doctor.* Check with your doctor immediately if you experience any of the following:

- seizure, changes in blood pressure, irregular heart rate, shortness of breath, problems with urination,(difficult or painful urination; unable to urinate), confusion, extreme sedation, excitation or mania, severe skin sensitivity to sunlight (burning or blistering), extreme constipation, yellow skin or eyes

Some side effects appear when you first start taking desipramine and go away for most people. If the following side effects continue, contact your doctor.

- stimulation, anxiety, insomnia, dizziness, blurred vision, dry mouth, mild to moderate constipation, increased appetite, weight gain, breast enlargement (men or women), discharge from the breast, sexual problems, hand tremor, persistent sore throat

Drug Interactions
Desipramine can adversely interact with the following frequently prescribed medications:

- cimetidine (Tagamet)—can cause high desipramine levels
- SSRI antidepressants—can cause high desipramine levels
- MAOI antidepressants—severe reaction causing dangerously high blood pressure, high body temperature, seizures, or death
- clonidine—if clonidine is being taken for high blood pressure, desipramine may cause clonidine to work less well
- antipsychotics—may increase certain neurologic side effects

- thyroid hormones—increased effects of both, especially excitation and changes in the heart rate or rhythm
- drugs used during surgery—can cause increased blood pressure. Make sure your doctors are aware of upcoming planned surgeries

MEDICAL CONSIDERATIONS

If you have any of the following medical conditions, make sure your doctor is aware of it.

- liver disease or alcoholism—desipramine levels may be higher than expected
- kidney disease—desipramine levels may be higher than expected
- glaucoma—desipramine can increase pressure inside the eye
- heart problems—some heart problems can be worsened by desipramine. It should not be taken by someone who has had a recent heart attack
- urinary retention, prostate enlargement—urination may be more difficult
- seizure disorder—desipramine can lower seizure threshold
- diabetes mellitus (sugar diabetes)—blood sugar levels may be affected
- thyroid disorders—desipramine may cause increased heart rate

---

Drug Name: DIAZEPAM   (dye-A-ze-pam)

Drug Category: Antianxiety medicine
Requires prescription, controlled substance, moderate potential for abuse

Commonly Used Brand-Name Products	
Tablets Valium (and generic) 2 mg, 5 mg and 10 mg **Capsules, sustained release** Valrelease 15 mg	**Liquid** Valium (and generic) 5 mg/ml (concentrate) Generic, 5 mg/teaspoonful **Injection** Valium (and generic) 5 mg/ml

GENERAL INFORMATION

Highly effective in treating anxiety and nervousness. Also used to treat panic disorder, and symptoms of alcohol withdrawal.

Before Taking this Medication

Talk to your doctor about the benefits and risks associated with diazepam. Make sure you understand how to take it safely and effectively. Make sure your doctor has the following information in detail:

- any allergic or bad reactions you have had to diazepam or any other medication
- all prescription and over-the-counter medicines you are taking
- your complete medical history
- if you are pregnant, could be pregnant, or are planning a pregnancy in the near future, diazepam has not been shown to be absolutely safe
- if you are breast-feeding, diazepam can pass into breast milk and affect the baby

DOSAGE

<u>Adults:</u> 2 to 10 mg 2 to 4 times a day (regular tablets or liquid forms) or 15–30 mg daily (long-acting capsule).

<u>Older adults</u> are more susceptible to side effects and generally require lower dosages.

<u>Children over 6 months:</u> When used in children, dosage is based on body weight.

<u>Children under 6 months:</u> Dosages in this age group have not been established.

DIRECTIONS FOR PROPER USE

- *Take exactly as prescribed. Do not take more or less than prescribed. Diazepam levels that are too high can cause serious toxicity.*
- If stomach upset occurs, diazepam may be taken with food.
- If you take diazepam regularly for an extended period of time, do not stop taking it unless told to do so by your doctor. It may be necessary to gradually reduce the dose of diazepam before stopping completely.
- If you taking the concentrated liquid form, mix your dose in water or fruit juice, or applesauce or pudding, before taking. Measure the dose carefully. Take immediately, do not save for later use.
- If you miss a dose of the tablet or a liquid form, take it as soon as possible. However, if the missed dose is within 6 hours of your next dose, skip the missed dose and resume with your next scheduled dose.

- **If you are taking the long-acting capsule form:**
  - Swallow the capsule whole. Do not crush, open, or chew it.
  - If you miss a dose, take it as soon as possible. However, if the missed dose is within 8 hours of your next dose, skip the missed dose and resume with your next scheduled dose.
  - Long-acting capsules are not interchangeable with regular diazepam tablets or liquid forms.

PRECAUTIONS
Alcohol should be avoided while taking diazepam.

Side Effects
Not all side effects will occur. Many side effects will diminish with time. *However, some side effects may be warning signs of toxicity and will require attention from your doctor.* Check with your doctor immediately if you experience any of the following:

- confusion, severe drowsiness, slurred speech, severe weakness, unusual thoughts, shortness of breath, excitement, hyperactivity

Some side effects appear when you first start taking diazepam and go away for most people. If the following side effects continue, contact your doctor.

- dizziness, light-headedness, drowsiness, blurred vision, stomach problems

Drug Interactions
Diazepam can adversely interact with the following frequently prescribed medications:

- cimetidine (Tagamet)—can cause high diazepam levels
- disulfiram (Antabuse)—can cause high diazepam levels
- birth control pills—can cause high diazepam levels
- alcohol and other drugs that depress certain functions of the nervous system, when combined with diazepam, can cause extreme drowsiness and slowed reaction times. Examples of these medicines are antihistamines, narcotics, and barbiturates.
- levodopa—decreased effectiveness of levodopa

MEDICAL CONSIDERATIONS
If you have any of the following medical conditions, make sure your doctor is aware of it.

- liver disease or alcoholism—diazepam levels may be higher than expected
- kidney disease—diazepam levels may be higher than expected

- drug dependence or alcohol dependence—dependence on diazepam may occur
- seizure disorder—stopping diazepam abruptly may cause seizures
- chronic lung disease—diazepam may make breathing more difficult

---

Drug Name: DOXEPIN   (dox-e-pin)

Drug Category: Antidepressant, tricyclic
Requires prescription

Commonly Used Brand-Name Products
Capsules
Sinequan, Adapin (and generic) 10 mg, 25 mg, 50 mg, 75 mg, 100 mg, 150 mg
Solution
Doxepin 10 mg/ml

GENERAL INFORMATION
Highly effective in treating major depression and the depressed phase of bipolar disorder. Very effective in treating panic disorder. Also used to treat certain chronic pain disorders, such as migraine headache and diabetic neuropathy. Sometimes given in low doses to help with insomnia.

Before Taking this Medication
Talk to your doctor about the benefits and risks associated with doxepin. Make sure you understand how to take it safely and effectively. Make sure your doctor has the following information in detail:

- any allergic or bad reactions you have had to doxepin or any other medication
- all prescription and over-the-counter medicines you are taking
- your complete medical history
- if you are pregnant, could be pregnant, or are planning a pregnancy in the near future, doxepin has not been shown to be absolutely safe.
- if you are breast-feeding, doxepin can pass into breast milk and affect the baby

DOSAGE

The starting dose of doxepin will be low and gradually be increased.

<u>Adults:</u>

<u>Depression, panic disorder:</u> Starting dose 25–50 mg at bedtime. Increased to 75–300 mg at bedtime over 2 to 3 weeks.

<u>Insomnia:</u> 10–50 mg at bedtime.

<u>Chronic pain syndromes:</u> 25–100 mg daily.

<u>Adolescents:</u> Adolescents may be more susceptible to heart-related side effects. Blood levels and heart function should be monitored.

<u>Children under 12:</u> Safe use and dosages in this age group have not been established. Children are more susceptible to serious heart-related side effects. Blood levels and heart function should be monitored.

<u>Older adults</u> are more susceptible to side effects and generally require lower dosages.

DIRECTIONS FOR PROPER USE

- *Take exactly as prescribed. Do not take more or less than prescribed. Accidental or intended overdoses of doxepin are potentially fatal.*
- If you miss a bedtime dose, do not take it the next morning. It may make you drowsy. Do not double doses.
- If you take the liquid form of doxepin, it must be mixed in liquid before taking. Use the dropper that comes with the original bottle. See below for specific list of acceptable liquids.
- The liquid form of doxepin must be mixed in 4 oz. of water, milk, citrus fruit juice, or tomato or prune juice before taking. **Do not** mix in grape or carbonated beverages. Take immediately after mixing. Do not store for later use.
- It may take several weeks before you feel the full benefits.
- Laboratory tests may be done to determine if the amount of doxepin in your bloodstream is in the correct range.
- Do not abruptly stop taking doxepin unless instructed to do so by your doctor. Gradually reducing the dose can help prevent mood changes, headache, or diarrhea.

PRECAUTIONS

Alcohol can cause changes in mood and may interfere with doxepin's effectiveness. *Alcohol should be avoided while taking doxepin.*

Side Effects

Not all side effects will occur. Many side effects will diminish with time. *However, some side effects may require attention from your doctor.* Check with your doctor immediately if you experience any of the following:

- seizure, changes in blood pressure, irregular heart rate, shortness of breath, problems with urination, (difficult or painful urination; unable to urinate), confusion, extreme sedation, excitation or mania, severe skin sensitivity to sunlight (burning or blistering), extreme constipation, yellow skin or eyes

Some side effects appear when you first start taking doxepin and go away for most people. If the following side effects continue, contact your doctor.

- dizziness, blurred vision, dry mouth, mild to moderate constipation, increased appetite, weight gain, breast enlargement (men or women), discharge from the breast, sexual problems, hand tremor, persistent sore throat

Drug Interactions

Doxepin can adversely interact with the following frequently prescribed medications:

- cimetidine (Tagamet)—can cause high doxepin levels
- SSRI antidepressants—can cause high doxepin levels
- MAOI antidepressants—severe reaction causing dangerously high blood pressure, high body temperature, seizures, or death
- clonidine—if clonidine is being taken for high blood pressure, doxepin may cause clonidine to work less well
- antipsychotics—may increase certain neurologic side effects
- thyroid hormones—increased effects of both, especially excitation and changes in heart rate or rhythm
- drugs used during surgery—can cause increased blood pressure. Make sure your doctors are aware of upcoming planned surgeries

MEDICAL CONSIDERATIONS

If you have any of the following medical conditions, make sure your doctor is aware of it.

- liver disease or alcoholism—doxepin levels may be higher than expected
- kidney disease—doxepin levels may be higher than expected
- glaucoma—doxepin can increase pressure inside the eye

- heart problems—some heart problems can be worsened by doxepin. It should not be taken by someone who has had a recent heart attack
- urinary retention, prostate enlargement—urination may become more difficult
- seizure disorder—doxepin can lower seizure threshold
- diabetes mellitus (sugar diabetes)—blood sugar levels may be affected
- thyroid disorders—doxepin may cause increased heart rate

Drug Name: ESTAZOLAM   (es-TAZ-o-lam)

Drug Category: Insomnia medicine
Requires prescription, controlled substance, moderate potential for abuse

Commonly Used Brand-Name Products
Tablets   ProSom, 1 mg and 2 mg

GENERAL INFORMATION
Highly effective in treating insomnia.

Before Taking this Medication
Talk to your doctor about the benefits and risks associated with estazolam. Make sure you understand how to take it safely and effectively. You and your family members should be very familiar with the side effects and signs of having too much estazolam in your system. Make sure your doctor has the following information in detail:
- any allergic or bad reactions you have had to estazolam or any other medication
- all prescription and over-the-counter medicines you are taking
- your complete medical history
- if you are pregnant, could be pregnant, or are planning a pregnancy in the near future, estazolam should not be taken
- if you are breast-feeding, estazolam can pass into breast milk and affect the baby

DOSAGE
<u>Adults:</u> 1 mg to 2 mg at bedtime.

<u>Older adults</u> are more susceptible to side effects and generally require lower dosages.

<u>Children under 18:</u> Safe use has not been established in this age group.

DIRECTIONS FOR PROPER USE

- *Take exactly as prescribed. Do not take more or less than prescribed. Estazolam levels that are too high can cause serious toxicity.*
- If you take estazolam regularly for an extended period of time, do not stop taking it unless told to do so by your doctor. It may be necessary to gradually reduce the dose before stopping completely.
- If you miss a dose, take it as soon as possible if it is within one hour of the scheduled time. However, estazolam should be taken only if you are sure you will get a full night's sleep of at least 7 to 8 hours.

PRECAUTIONS

Alcohol should be avoided while taking estazolam.

Side Effects

Not all side effects will occur. Many side effects will diminish with time. *However, some side effects may be warning signs of toxicity and will require attention from your doctor.* Check with your doctor immediately if you experience any of the following:

- confusion, severe drowsiness, slurred speech, severe weakness, unusual thoughts, shortness of breath, excitement, hyperactivity

Some side effects appear when you first start taking estazolam and go away for most people. If the following side effects continue, contact your doctor.

- dizziness, light-headedness, daytime drowsiness, blurred vision

Drug Interactions

Estazolam can adversely interact with the following frequently prescribed medications:

- cimetidine (Tagamet)—can cause high estazolam levels
- disulfiram (Antabuse)—can cause high estazolam levels
- birth control pills—can cause high estazolam levels
- alcohol and other drugs that depress certain functions of the nervous system, when combined with estazolam, can cause extreme drowsiness and slowed reaction times. Examples of these medicines are antihistamines, narcotics, and barbiturates.

- levodopa—decreased effectiveness of levodopa

MEDICAL CONSIDERATIONS

If you have any of the following medical conditions, make sure your doctor is aware of it.

- liver disease or alcoholism—estazolam levels may be higher than expected
- kidney disease—estazolam levels may be higher than expected
- drug dependence or alcohol dependence—dependence on estazolam may occur
- seizure disorder—stopping estazolam abruptly may cause seizures
- chronic lung disease—estazolam may make breathing more difficult

---

Drug Name: FLUOXETINE   (flu-OX-a-teen)

Drug Category: Antidepressant, SSRI
(serotonin specific reuptake inhibitor)
Requires prescription

Commonly Used Brand-Name Products
Capsules
Prozac 10 mg, 20 mg
Solution
Prozac 20 mg/5ml

GENERAL INFORMATION

Highly effective in treating major depression, the depressed phase of bipolar disorder, and obsessive compulsive disorder (OCD). Effective in treating panic disorder. May be useful in treating bulimia. May be used to treat attention deficit hyperactivity disorder, especially in adults.

Before Taking this Medication

Talk to your doctor about the benefits and risks associated with fluoxetine. Make sure you understand how to take fluoxetine safely and effectively. Make sure your doctor has the following information in detail:

- any allergic or bad reactions you have had to fluoxetine or any other medication

- all prescription and over-the-counter medicines you are taking
- your complete medical history
- if you are pregnant, could be pregnant, or are planning a pregnancy in the near future, fluoxetine has not been shown to be absolutely safe
- if you are breast-feeding, fluoxetine can pass into breast milk and affect the baby

DOSAGE
Adults and adolescents:
>Depression, panic disorder, bulimia: 10–40 mg daily. Sometimes higher doses are required. Dosage increases should not be more often than every 4 weeks.
>OCD: 20–80 mg daily.

Children under 12: Safe use and dosages in this age group have not been established.

Older adults are more susceptible to side effects and generally require lower dosages.

DIRECTIONS FOR PROPER USE
- *Take exactly as prescribed. Do not take more or less than prescribed.*
- Fluoxetine may be taken with food to lessen stomach upset.
- If you miss a dose, do not try to make it up. Wait and take your next scheduled dose. Do not double doses.
- It may take several weeks (up to 5 weeks) before you feel the full benefits.
- Do not abruptly stop taking fluoxetine unless instructed to do so by your doctor.

PRECAUTIONS
Alcohol can cause changes in mood and may interfere with fluoxetine's effectiveness. *Alcohol should be avoided while taking fluoxetine.*

Side Effects
Not all side effects will occur. Many side effects will diminish with time. *However, some side effects may require attention from your doctor.* Check with your doctor immediately if you experience any of the following:

- skin rash or hives, shortness of breath, chills or fever, swelling of the hands or feet, seizures, sore throat

Some side effects appear when you first start taking fluoxetine and go away for most people. If the following side effects continue, contact your doctor.

- stimulation, anxiety, insomnia, dizziness, sexual problems, sweating, blurred vision, dry mouth, mild to moderate constipation, change in appetite, change in weight, hand tremor, headache

Drug Interactions

Fluoxetine can adversely interact with the following frequently prescribed medications:

- anticoagulants (blood thinners)—the effect of the anticoagulant can be increased
- some nonsedating antihistamines—cardiac (heart) toxicity
- diet pills—severe reaction causing dangerously high blood pressure, high body temperature, seizures, or death
- products containing l-tryptophan—severe reaction causing dangerously high blood pressure, high body temperature, seizures, or death
- cimetidine (Tagamet)—can cause high fluoxetine levels
- TCA antidepressants—can cause high TCA levels
- MAOI antidepressants—severe reaction causing dangerously high blood pressure, high body temperature, seizures, or death
- antipsychotics—may increase certain neurologic side effects
- lithium—increased lithium levels may cause confusion, dizziness, tremor
- anticonvulsants—increased anticonvulsant levels or decreased fluoxetine levels

MEDICAL CONSIDERATIONS

If you have any of the following medical conditions, make sure your doctor is aware of it.

- liver disease or alcoholism—fluoxetine levels may be higher than expected
- kidney disease—fluoxetine levels may be higher than expected
- seizure disorder—fluoxetine can lower seizure threshold
- diabetes mellitus (sugar diabetes)—blood sugar levels may be affected

Drug Name: FLUPHENAZINE   (flew-FEN-a-zeen)

Drug Category: Neuroleptic; Antipsychotic

Requires prescription

Commonly Used Brand-Name Products	
Tablets	**Injection**
Prolixin, Permitil	Prolixin (and generic),
(and generic), 1 mg, 2.5 mg,	2.5 mg/ml
5 mg, 10 mg	**Injection, long-acting**
Liquid	Prolixin decanoate
Prolixin, Permitil	(and generic) 25 mg/ml
(and generic) solution	Prolixin enanthate
5 mg/ml (contains alcohol)	25 mg/ml

GENERAL INFORMATION

Highly effective in treating psychotic symptoms such as hallucinations and delusions. These symptoms occur in schizophrenia, schizoaffective disorder, bipolar disorder or major depression with psychotic features. Can also be used for the short-term management of aggressive, out-of-control behaviors, or feelings of anger and rage. Can be used to help with symptoms of anxiety and insomnia.

Before Taking this Medication

Talk to your doctor about the benefits and risks associated with fluphenazine. Make sure you understand how to take it safely and effectively. You and your family members should be very familiar with the side effects. Make sure your doctor has the following information in detail:

- any allergic or bad reactions you have had to fluphenazine or any other medication
- all prescription and over-the-counter medicines you are taking
- your complete medical history
- if you are pregnant, could be pregnant, or are planning a pregnancy in the near future, fluphenazine has not been shown to be absolutely safe
- if you are breast-feeding, fluphenazine can pass into breast milk and affect the baby

DOSAGE

Adults and adolescents:

<u>Psychotic symptoms:</u> 5–80 mg daily. There is a wide effective dosage range.

<u>Anxiety and insomnia:</u> 2.5–5 mg daily, usually at bedtime, but in extreme anxiety can be given during waking hours.

<u>Older adults</u> are more susceptible to side effects and generally require lower dosages.

<u>Children under 12:</u> Dosages in this age group have not been established.

DIRECTIONS FOR PROPER USE

- *Take exactly as prescribed. Do not take more or less than prescribed.*
- If you take the solution form, avoid contact of the skin with the medicine. Irritation can result by the medicine coming into contact with skin. Do not use the liquid form if it becomes very discolored (dark yellow) or has a sediment at the bottom of the bottle.
- The long-acting shot form of fluphenazine can have an effect up to 4 weeks after the shot is given.
- If you miss a dose, take it as soon as possible. However, if the missed dose is within 4 hours of your next dose, skip the missed dose and resume with your next scheduled dose.
- It may take several weeks before you feel the full benefits.

PRECAUTIONS

Alcohol should be avoided while taking fluphenazine.

Side Effects

Not all side effects will occur. Many side effects will diminish with time. *However, some side effects may be warning signs of toxicity and will require attention from your doctor.* Check with your doctor immediately if you experience any of the following:

- seizure, high fever, fast or irregular heartbeat, very low blood pressure, faintness, any abnormal movements of the mouth, tongue, neck, arms or legs, difficulty speaking or swallowing, imbalance or difficulty walking normally, severe muscle stiffness, discoloration of the skin or eyes, confusion, significant drowsiness, restlessness, difficulty urinating, sexual problems, vomiting, diarrhea, unusual bruising or bleeding, severe skin reaction to sunlight (burning or blistering), severe constipation, breast pain or enlargement

Some side effects appear when you first start taking fluphenazine and go away for most people. If the following side effects continue, contact your doctor.

- dry mouth, mild to moderate constipation, dizziness, hand tremor, stuffy nose, weight gain

Drug Interactions
Fluphenazine can adversely interact with the following frequently prescribed medications:

- lithium—increased neurologic side effects
- levodopa—decreased effectiveness of levodopa
- amphetamines—increased psychotic symptoms are possible
- anticonvulsants—decreased fluphenazine levels
- tricyclic antidepressants—increased TCA levels

MEDICAL CONSIDERATIONS
If you have any of the following medical conditions, make sure your doctor is aware of it.

- kidney disease—fluphenazine levels may be higher than expected
- liver disease—fluphenazine levels may be higher than expected
- heart problems—some heart problems can be worsened by fluphenazine
- seizure disorder—fluphenazine can lower seizure threshold
- urinary retention, prostate enlargement—urination may be more difficult
- glaucoma—fluphenazine can increase pressure inside the eye
- Parkinson's disease—some Parkinson's symptoms may be worsened
- breast cancer—may increase risk of cancer progression

Drug Name: FLURAZEPAM   (flur-AZ-e-pam)

Drug Category: Insomnia medicine
Requires prescription, controlled substance, moderate potential for abuse

Commonly Used Brand-Name Products
Capsules
Dalmane (and generic) 15 mg and 30 mg

GENERAL INFORMATION
Highly effective in treating insomnia.

Before Taking this Medication
Talk to your doctor about the benefits and risks associated with flurazepam. Make sure you understand how to take it safely and effectively. You and your family members should be very familiar with the side effects and signs of having too much flurazepam in your system. Make sure your doctor has the following information in detail:

- any allergic or bad reactions you have had to flurazepam or any other medication
- all prescription and over-the-counter medicines you are taking
- your complete medical history
- if you are pregnant, could be pregnant, or are planning a pregnancy in the near future, flurazepam should not be taken
- if you are breast-feeding, flurazepam can pass into breast milk and affect the baby

DOSAGE
Adults: 15 mg to 30 mg at bedtime.

Older adults are more susceptible to side effects and generally require lower dosages.

Children under 18: Safe use has not been established in this age group.

DIRECTIONS FOR PROPER USE
- *Take exactly as prescribed. Do not take more or less than prescribed. Flurazepam levels that are too high can cause serious toxicity.*
- If you will be taking flurazepam regularly for an extended period of time, do not stop taking it unless told to do so by your doctor. It may be necessary to gradually reduce the dose before stopping completely.
- If you miss a dose, take it as soon as possible if it is within one hour of the scheduled time. However, flurazepam should be taken only if you are sure you will get a full night's sleep of at least 7 to 8 hours.

PRECAUTIONS
Alcohol should be avoided while taking flurazepam.

Side Effects
Not all side effects will occur. Many side effects will diminish with time. *However, some side effects may be warning signs of*

toxicity and will require attention from your doctor. Check with your doctor immediately if you experience any of the following:

- confusion, severe drowsiness, slurred speech, severe weakness, unusual thoughts, shortness of breath, excitement, hyperactivity

Some side effects appear when you first start taking flurazepam and go away for most people. If the following side effects continue, contact your doctor.

- dizziness, light-headedness, daytime drowsiness, blurred vision

Drug Interactions

Flurazepam can adversely interact with the following frequently prescribed medications:

- cimetidine (Tagamet)—can cause high flurazepam levels
- disulfiram (Antabuse)—can cause high flurazepam levels
- birth control pills—can cause high flurazepam levels
- alcohol and other drugs that depress certain functions of the nervous system, when combined with flurazepam, can cause extreme drowsiness and slowed reaction times. Examples of these medicines are antihistamines, narcotics, and barbiturates.
- levodopa—decreased effectiveness of levodopa

MEDICAL CONSIDERATIONS

If you have any of the following medical conditions, make sure your doctor is aware of it.

- liver disease or alcoholism—flurazepam levels may be higher than expected
- kidney disease—flurazepam levels may be higher than expected
- drug dependence or alcohol dependence—dependence on flurazepam may occur
- seizure disorder—stopping flurazepam abruptly may cause seizures
- chronic lung disease—flurazepam may make breathing more difficult

---

Drug Name: FLUVOXAMINE   (flu-VOX-a-meen)

Drug Category: Antidepressant, SSRI
(serotonin specific reuptake inhibitor)
Requires prescription

Commonly Used Brand-Name Products
Tablets Luvox 50 mg, 100 mg

GENERAL INFORMATION
Highly effective in treating obsessive compulsive disorder (OCD). Also effective in treating major depression.

Before Taking this Medication
Talk to your doctor about the benefits and risks associated with fluvoxamine. Make sure you understand how to take it safely and effectively. Make sure your doctor has the following information in detail:

- any allergic or bad reactions you have had to fluvoxamine or any other medication
- all prescription and over-the-counter medicines you are taking
- your complete medical history
- if you are pregnant, could be pregnant, or are planning a pregnancy in the near future, fluvoxamine has not been shown to be absolutely safe.
- if you are breast-feeding, fluvoxamine can pass into breast milk and affect the baby

DOSAGE
<u>Adults and adolescents:</u> 50–300 mg daily. The starting dose of fluvoxamine will be low and gradually be increased depending on your response and the side effects.

<u>Older adults</u> are more susceptible to side effects and generally require lower dosages.

<u>Children under 16:</u> Safe use and dosages in this age group have not been established

DIRECTIONS FOR PROPER USE
- *Take exactly as prescribed. Do not take more or less than prescribed.*
- Fluvoxamine may be taken with food to lessen stomach upset.
- If you miss a dose, do not try to make it up. Wait and take your next scheduled dose. Do not double doses.
- It may take several weeks before you feel the full benefits.
- Do not abruptly stop taking fluvoxamine unless instructed to do so by your doctor.

PRECAUTIONS

Alcohol can cause changes in mood and may interfere with fluvoxamine's effectiveness. *Alcohol should be avoided while taking fluvoxamine.*

Side Effects

Not all side effects will occur. Many side effects will diminish with time. *However, some side effects may require attention from your doctor.* Check with your doctor immediately if you experience any of the following:

- skin rash or hives, shortness of breath, chills or fever, swelling of the hands or feet, seizures, sore throat

Some side effects appear when you first start taking fluvoxamine and go away for most people. If the following side effects continue, contact your doctor.

- fatigue, drowsiness, dizziness, sexual problems, sweating, blurred vision, dry mouth, mild to moderate constipation, change in appetite, change in weight, hand tremor, headache

Drug Interactions

Fluvoxamine can adversely interact with the following frequently prescribed medications:

- anticoagulants (blood thinners)—the effect of the anticoagulant can be increased
- some nonsedating antihistamines—cardiac (heart) toxicity
- diet pills—severe reaction causing dangerously high blood pressure, high body temperature, seizures, or death
- products containing l-tryptophan—severe reaction causing dangerously high blood pressure, high body temperature, seizures, or death
- cimetidine (Tagamet)—can cause high fluvoxamine levels
- TCA antidepressants—can cause high TCA levels
- MAOI antidepressants—severe reaction causing dangerously high blood pressure, high body temperature, seizures, or death
- antipsychotics—may increase certain neurologic side effects
- lithium—increased lithium levels may cause confusion, dizziness, tremor
- anticonvulsants—increased anticonvulsant levels or decreased fluvoxamine levels

MEDICAL CONSIDERATIONS

If you have any of the following medical conditions, make sure your doctor is aware of it.

- liver disease or alcoholism—fluvoxamine levels may be higher than expected
- kidney disease—fluvoxamine levels may be higher than expected
- seizure disorder—fluvoxamine can lower seizure threshold
- diabetes mellitus (sugar diabetes)—blood sugar levels may be affected

---

Drug Name: HALAZEPAM   (hal-AZ-e-pam)

Drug Category: Antianxiety medicine
Requires prescription, controlled substance, moderate potential for abuse

Commonly Used Brand-Name Products
Tablets Paxipam 20 mg and 40 mg

GENERAL INFORMATION
Highly effective in treating anxiety and nervousness.

Before Taking this Medication
Talk to your doctor about the benefits and risks associated with halazepam. Make sure you understand how to take it safely and effectively. You and your family members should be very familiar with the side effects and signs of having too much halazepam in your system. Make sure your doctor has the following information in detail:

- any allergic or bad reactions you have had to halazepam or any other medication
- all prescription and over-the-counter medicines you are taking
- your complete medical history
- if you are pregnant, could be pregnant, or are planning a pregnancy in the near future, halazepam should not be taken
- if you are breast-feeding, halazepam can pass into breast milk and affect the baby

DOSAGE
The starting dose of halazepam will be low and gradually be increased depending on your response and the side effects.
Adults:
   Anxiety: 20 to 40 mg up to 4 times a day.

<u>Older adults</u> are more susceptible to side effects and generally require lower dosages.

<u>Children under 18:</u> Safe use has not been established in this age group.

DIRECTIONS FOR PROPER USE

- *Take exactly as prescribed. Do not take more or less than prescribed. Halazepam levels that are too high can cause serious toxicity.*
- If you take halazepam regularly for an extended period of time, do not stop taking it unless told to do so by your doctor. It may be necessary to gradually reduce the dose before stopping completely.
- If you miss a dose, take it as soon as possible. However, if the missed dose is within 4 hours of your next dose, skip the missed dose, and resume with your next scheduled dose.

PRECAUTIONS

Alcohol should be avoided while taking halazepam.

Side Effects

Not all side effects will occur. Many side effects will diminish with time. *However, some side effects may be warning signs of toxicity and will require attention from your doctor.* Check with your doctor immediately if you experience any of the following:

- confusion, severe drowsiness, slurred speech, severe weakness, unusual thoughts, shortness of breath, excitement, hyperactivity

Some side effects appear when you first start taking halazepam and go away for most people. If the following side effects continue, contact your doctor.

- dizziness, light-headedness, drowsiness, blurred vision, stomach problems

Drug Interactions

Halazepam can adversely interact with the following frequently prescribed medications:

- cimetidine (Tagamet)—can cause high halazepam levels
- disulfiram (Antabuse)—can cause high halazepam levels
- birth control pills—can cause high halazepam levels
- alcohol and other drugs that depress certain functions of the nervous system, when combined with halazepam, can cause extreme drowsiness and slowed reaction times. Examples of these medicines are antihistamines, narcotics, and barbiturates.

- levodopa—decreased effectiveness of levodopa

MEDICAL CONSIDERATIONS

If you have any of the following medical conditions, make sure your doctor is aware of it.

- liver disease or alcoholism—halazepam levels may be higher than expected
- kidney disease—halazepam levels may be higher than expected
- drug dependence or alcohol dependence—dependence on halazepam may occur
- seizure disorder—stopping halazepam abruptly may cause seizures
- chronic lung disease—halazepam may make breathing more difficult

---

Drug Name: HALOPERIDOL   (ha-lo-PER-i-dol)

Drug Category: Neuroleptic; Antipsychotic
Requires prescription

Commonly Used Brand-Name Products	
Tablets	**Injection**
Haldol (and generic) 0.5 mg, 1 mg, 2.5 mg, 5 mg, 10 mg, 20 mg	Haldol (and generic) 5 mg/ml
Liquid	**Injection, long-acting**
Haldol (and generic) solution 2 mg/ml (contains alcohol)	Haldol decanoate 50 mg/ml, 100 mg/ml

GENERAL INFORMATION

Highly effective in treating psychotic symptoms, such as hallucinations and delusions. These symptoms occur in schizophrenia, schizoaffective disorder, bipolar disorder or major depression with psychotic features. Also effective in treating Tourette's syndrome, to help reduce motor tics and vocalizations. Can be used for the short-term management of aggressive, out-of-control behaviors or feelings of anger and rage. Haloperidol is also used to help with symptoms of anxiety and insomnia, and to control psychotic symptoms in dementing illnesses.

Before Taking this Medication

Talk to your doctor about the benefits and risks associated with haloperidol. Make sure you understand how to take it safely and effectively. You and your family members should be very familiar with the side effects. Make sure your doctor has the following information in detail:

- any allergic or bad reactions you have had to haloperidol or any other medication
- all prescription and over-the-counter medicines you are taking
- your complete medical history
- if you are pregnant, could be pregnant, or are planning a pregnancy in the near future, haloperidol has not been shown to be absolutely safe.
- if you are breast-feeding, haloperidol can pass into breast milk and affect the baby

DOSAGE

Adults and adolescents:

Psychotic symptoms, Tourette's syndrome: 5–80 mg daily. There is a wide effective dosage range.

Anxiety and insomnia: 2.5–5 mg daily, usually at bedtime, but in extreme anxiety can be given during waking hours.

Older adults are more susceptible to side effects and generally require lower dosages.

Children 3-12: Dosages are based on body weight.

Children under 3: Dosages in this age group have not been established.

DIRECTIONS FOR PROPER USE

- *Take exactly as prescribed. Do not take more or less than prescribed.*
- The liquid form of haloperidol should not be mixed in coffee, tea, or juice. Mix it in water and take immediately.
- If you take the solution form, avoid contact of the skin with the medicine. Irritation can result by the medicine coming in contact with skin. Do not use the liquid form if it becomes very discolored (dark yellow) or has a sediment at the bottom of the bottle.
- The long-acting shot form of haloperidol may have an effect for up to 6 weeks.

- If you miss a dose, take it as soon as possible. However, if the missed dose is within 4 hours of your next dose, skip the missed dose and resume with your next scheduled dose.
- It may take several weeks before you feel the full benefits.

PRECAUTIONS
Alcohol should be avoided while taking haloperidol.

Side Effects
Not all side effects will occur. Many side effects will diminish with time. *However, some side effects may be warning signs of toxicity and will require attention from your doctor.* Check with your doctor immediately if you experience any of the following:

- seizure, high fever, fast or irregular heartbeat, very low blood pressure, faintness, any abnormal movements of the mouth, tongue, neck, arms or legs, difficulty speaking or swallowing, imbalance or difficulty walking normally, severe muscle stiffness, discoloration of the skin or eyes, confusion, significant drowsiness, restlessness, difficulty urinating, sexual problems, vomiting, diarrhea, unusual bruising or bleeding, severe skin reaction to sunlight (burning or blistering), severe constipation, breast pain or enlargement

Some side effects appear when you first start taking haloperidol and go away for most people. If the following side effects continue, contact your doctor.

- dry mouth, mild to moderate constipation, dizziness, hand tremor, stuffy nose, weight gain

Drug Interactions
Haloperidol can adversely interact with the following frequently prescribed medications:

- lithium—increased neurologic side effects
- levodopa—decreased effectiveness of levodopa
- amphetamines—increased psychotic symptoms are possible
- anticonvulsants—decreased haloperidol levels
- tricyclic antidepressants—increased TCA levels

MEDICAL CONSIDERATIONS
If you have any of the following medical conditions, make sure your doctor is aware of it.

- kidney disease—haloperidol levels may be higher than expected
- liver disease—haloperidol levels may be higher than expected

- heart problems—some heart problems can be worsened by haloperidol
- seizure disorder—haloperidol can lower seizure threshold
- urinary retention, prostate enlargement—urination may be more difficult
- glaucoma—haloperidol can increase pressure inside the eye
- Parkinson's disease—some Parkinson's symptoms may be worsened
- breast cancer—may increase risk of cancer progression

Drug Name: IMIPRAMINE   (im-IP-ra-meen)
Drug Category: Antidepressant, tricyclic
Requires prescription

Commonly Used Brand-Name Products
Tablets
Tofranil (and generic) 10 mg, 25 mg, 50 mg
Capsules, as pamoate
Tofranil PM 75 mg, 100 mg, 125 mg, 150 mg
Injection
Tofranil 12.5 mg/ml

GENERAL INFORMATION
Highly effective in treating major depression and the depressed phase of bipolar disorder. Very effective in treating panic disorder. Also used to treat attention deficit hyperactivity disorder, especially in adults, and certain chronic pain disorders, such as migraine headache and diabetic neuropathy. In addition, imipramine is used to treat childhood enuresis (bedwetting).

Before Taking this Medication
Talk to your doctor about the benefits and risks associated with imipramine. Make sure you understand how to take it safely and effectively. Make sure your doctor has the following information in detail:

- any allergic or bad reactions you have had to imipramine or any other medication
- all prescription and over-the-counter medicines you are taking
- your complete medical history

- if you are pregnant, could be pregnant, or are planning a pregnancy in the near future, imipramine has not been shown to be absolutely safe.
- if you are breast-feeding, imipramine can pass into breast milk and affect the baby

DOSAGE

The starting dose of imipramine will be low and gradually be increased.

Adults:

Depression, panic disorder, ADHD: Starting dose 25–50 mg at bedtime. Increased to 75–300 mg at bedtime over 2 to 3 weeks.

Chronic pain syndromes: 25–100 mg daily.

Adolescents: Adolescents may be more susceptible to heart-related side effects. Blood levels and heart function should be monitored.

Children 6–12:

Depression: Official guidelines for safe use in depression for this age group have not been established. However, when used in this age group, dose is based on weight. Monitoring for blood levels and heart-related side effects is recommended.

Enuresis (in children at least 6 years of age): 25–50 mg at bedtime for children under 12. 25–75 mg at bedtime for children over 12. (½ the dose may be taken in midafternoon and ½ at bedtime for early in the night bedwetting).

Children under 6: Safe use and dosages in this age group have not been established. Children are more susceptible to serious heart-related side effects. Blood levels and heart function should be monitored.

Older adults are more susceptible to side effects and generally require lower dosages.

DIRECTIONS FOR PROPER USE

- *Take exactly as prescribed. Do not take more or less than prescribed. Accidental or intended overdoses of imipramine are potentially fatal.*
- Laboratory tests may be done to determine if the amount of imipramine in your bloodstream is in the correct range.
- If you miss a bedtime dose, do not take it the next morning. It may make you drowsy. Do not double doses.
- It may take several weeks before you feel the full benefits.
- Do not abruptly stop taking imipramine unless instructed to do so by your doctor. Gradually reducing the dose can help prevent mood changes, headache, or diarrhea.

PRECAUTIONS
Alcohol can cause changes in mood and may interfere with imipramine's effectiveness. *Alcohol should be avoided while taking imipramine.*

Side Effects
Not all side effects will occur. Many side effects will diminish with time. *However, some side effects may require attention from your doctor.* Check with your doctor immediately if you experience any of the following:

- seizure, changes in blood pressure, irregular heart rate, shortness of breath, problems with urination, (difficult or painful urination; unable to urinate), confusion, extreme sedation, excitation or mania, severe skin sensitivity to sunlight (burning or blistering), extreme constipation, yellow skin or eyes

Some side effects appear when you first start taking imipramine and go away for most people. If the following side effects continue, contact your doctor.

- stimulation, anxiety, insomnia, dizziness, blurred vision, dry mouth, mild to moderate constipation, increased appetite, weight gain, breast enlargement (men or women), discharge from the breast, sexual problems, hand tremor, persistent sore throat

Drug Interactions
Imipramine can adversely interact with the following frequently prescribed medications:

- cimetidine (Tagamet)—can cause high imipramine levels
- SSRI antidepressants—can cause high imipramine levels
- MAOI antidepressants—severe reaction causing dangerously high blood pressure, high body temperature, seizures, or death
- clonidine—if clonidine is being taken for high blood pressure, imipramine may cause clonidine to work less well
- antipsychotics—may increase certain neurologic side effects
- thyroid hormones—increased effects of both, especially excitation and changes in heart rate or rhythm
- drugs used during surgery—can cause increased blood pressure. Make sure your doctors are aware of upcoming planned surgeries

MEDICAL CONSIDERATIONS
Make sure your doctor is aware of it if you have any of the following medical conditions:

- liver disease, or alcoholism—imipramine levels may be higher than expected
- kidney disease—imipramine levels may be higher than expected
- glaucoma—imipramine can increase pressure inside the eye
- heart problems—some heart problems can be worsened by imipramine. It should not be taken by someone who has had a recent heart attack
- urinary retention, prostate enlargement—urination may become more difficult
- seizure disorder—imipramine can lower seizure threshold
- diabetes mellitus (sugar diabetes)—blood sugar levels may be affected
- thyroid disorders—imipramine may cause increased heart rate

---

Drug Name: LITHIUM (LITH-ee-um)
Drug Category: Mood stabilizer
Requires prescription

Commonly Used Brand-Name Products	
Tablets or capsules, as lithium carbonate (not extended release) Eskalith 300 mg tablets and 300 mg capsules Lithonate 300 mg capsules Lithotabs 300 mg tablets Various generic products available in 150 mg, 300 mg, and 600 mg tablets or capsules	**Extended release tablets, as lithium carbonate** Eskalith CR 450 mg tablets Lithobid 300 mg tablets **Syrup, as lithium citrate** Cibalith-S 300 mg/teaspoonful (sugar free)* Various generic products 300 mg/teaspoonful* * contains alcohol

GENERAL INFORMATION
Highly effective in treating bipolar disorder (manic-depressive disorder), especially acute manic and hypomanic phases. Lithium has also been shown to reduce the number and severity of subsequent episodes of both mania and depression. It can be used alone, or in combination with other mood stabilizers in severe cases. It is also used to treat schizoaffective disorder, usually in combination

with other medications called antipsychotics. Lithium can increase the effectiveness of antidepressants, and is sometimes given to people with major depression who have not responded to an anti-depressant alone. There is some evidence that it can help people who have significant problems with impulse control, by reducing anger or temper outbursts and aggressive behaviors.

Before Taking this Medication

Talk to your doctor about the benefits and risks associated with lithium. Make sure you understand how to take it safely and effectively. You and your family members should be very familiar with the side effects and signs of having too much lithium in your system. Make sure your doctor has the following information in detail:

- any allergic or bad reactions you have had to lithium or any other medication
- all prescription and over-the-counter medicines you are taking
- your complete medical history
- if you are pregnant, could be pregnant, or are planning a pregnancy in the near future, lithium should not be taken during pregnancy, especially the first three months. It can cause fetal heart and thyroid abnormalities
- if you are breast-feeding, lithium passes into breast milk and affects the baby

DOSAGE

The starting dose of lithium will be adjusted based on your response and blood levels. You may require more lithium during, and immediately following, an acute manic episode, than when your symptoms have stabilized.

Adults and adolescents:

    Acute mania: 300–600 mg 3 times daily. Maintenance dose: 300 mg 3 to 4 times daily.

Older adults are more susceptible to side effects and generally require lower dosages.

Children under 12: Dosages in this age group have not been established. However, when used in children, lithium dosage is based on body weight.

DIRECTIONS FOR PROPER USE

- *Take exactly as prescribed. Do not take more or less than prescribed. Lithum levels that are too high can cause serious toxicity.*

- Take lithium with meals or a snack. This will help relieve stomach upset or diarrhea.
- If you take the syrup form, mix your dose in fruit juice or another flavored beverage before taking.
- Drink lots of fluids throughout the day while taking lithium (2–3 quarts per day).
- Do not drink large amounts of coffee, tea, or colas. These beverages can cause increased urination and may also worsen hand tremor.
- Do not make drastic changes in your diet while taking lithium. It is important that your body not lose fluids or sodium when taking lithium. Use a normal amount of salt in your diet.
- Do not get dehydrated when taking lithium. Strenuous exercise, saunas, and hot weather can cause dehydration.
- If you miss a dose, take it as soon as possible. However, if the missed dose is within 4 hours of your next dose, skip the missed dose and resume with your next scheduled dose.
- If you are taking a long-acting form:
  - Swallow the tablet whole. Do not crush, split, or chew the tablet.
  - If you miss a dose, take it as soon as possible. However, if the missed dose is within 6 hours of your next dose, skip the missed dose and resume with your next scheduled dose.
  - Long-acting tablets are not interchangeable with regular lithium tablets, capsules, or liquid forms.
- It may take several weeks before you feel the full benefits.
- Laboratory tests are necessary to determine if the amount of lithium in your bloodstream is in the correct range.

PRECAUTIONS
Alcohol can cause changes in mood and may interfere with lithium's effectiveness. It can also cause increased urination and may affect lithium blood levels. *Alcohol should be avoided while taking lithium.*

Side Effects
Not all side effects will occur. Many side effects will diminish with time. *However, some side effects may be warning signs of toxicity and will require attention from your doctor.* Check with your doctor immediately if you experience any of the following:

- seizure, severe diarrhea, loss of appetite, severe nausea, muscle weakness, trembling, slurred speech, clumsiness, confusion, significant drowsiness, blurred vision, irregular heartbeat, difficulty breathing, swelling of the feet or hands

Some side effects appear when you first start taking lithium and go away for most people. If the following side effects continue, contact your doctor.

- mild hand tremor, mild nausea, mild diarrhea, thirst, increased frequency of urination, acne, weight gain, hair loss, sensitivity to cold

Drug Interactions

Lithium can adversely interact with the following frequently prescribed medications:

- diuretics (water pills)—can cause sodium loss leading to high lithium levels
- certain medications for high blood pressure
    calcium channel blockers—can cause increased lithium levels
    ACE inhibitors—can cause increased lithium levels
- pain relievers known as nonsteroidal antiinflammatory drugs (NSAIDs)—can cause lithium levels to increase
- antipsychotics—may increase certain neurologic side effects
- theophylline—can cause lithium levels to decrease

MEDICAL CONSIDERATIONS

If you have any of the following medical conditions, make sure your doctor is aware of it.

- kidney disease—lithium levels may be higher than expected
- thyroid disorders—lithium may worsen certain thyroid conditions
- heart problems—some heart problems can be worsened by lithium
- diabetes mellitus (sugar diabetes)—blood sugar levels can be increased
- dehydration—fluid and sodium may be lost, leading to increased lithium levels
- severe infection (with fever, sweating, diarrhea or vomiting)—can increase lithium levels
- Parkinson's disease—some Parkinson's symptoms may be worsened

Drug Name: LORAZEPAM   (lor-AZ-e-pam)

Drug Category: Antianxiety medicine
Requires prescription, controlled substance, moderate potential for abuse

Commonly Used Brand-Name Products
Tablets   Ativan (and generic) 0.5 mg, 1 mg and 2 mg   **Solution**   Ativan (and generic) 2 mg/ml   **Injection**   Ativan 2 mg/ml and 4 mg/ml

GENERAL INFORMATION
Highly effective in treating anxiety and nervousness. Also used to treat panic disorder and symptoms of alcohol withdrawal.

Before Taking this Medication
Talk to your doctor about the benefits and risks associated with lorazepam. Make sure you understand how to take it safely and effectively. You and your family members should be very familiar with the side effects and signs of having too much lorazepam in your system. Make sure your doctor has the following information in detail:

- any allergic or bad reactions you have had to lorazepam or any other medication
- all prescription and over-the-counter medicines you are taking
- your complete medical history
- if you are pregnant, could be pregnant, or are planning a pregnancy in the near future, lorazepam should not be taken.
- if you are breast-feeding, lorazepam can pass into breast milk and affect the baby

DOSAGE
Adults: 0.5 to 2 mg 2 to 3 times a day.
Older adults are more susceptible to side effects and generally require lower dosages.
Children under 12: When used in children, dosage is based on body weight.

DIRECTIONS FOR PROPER USE

- *Take exactly as prescribed. Do not take more or less than prescribed. Lorazepam levels that are too high can cause serious toxicity.*
- Lorazepam may be taken with food if stomach upset occurs.
- If you take lorazepam regularly for an extended period of time, do not stop taking it unless told to do so by your doctor. It may be necessary to gradually reduce the dose of lorazepam before stopping completely.
- If you miss a dose, take it as soon as possible. However, if the missed dose is within 4 hours of your next dose, skip the missed dose and resume with your next scheduled dose.
- If you are taking the liquid form, the dose should be mixed in water or soda, or applesauce or pudding.

PRECAUTIONS

Alcohol should be avoided while taking lorazepam.

Side Effects

Not all side effects will occur. Many side effects will diminish with time. *However, some side effects may be warning signs of toxicity and will require attention from your doctor.* Check with your doctor immediately if you experience any of the following:

- confusion, severe drowsiness, slurred speech, severe weakness, unusual thoughts, shortness of breath, excitement, hyperactivity

Some side effects appear when you first start taking lorazepam and go away for most people. If the following side effects continue, contact your doctor.

- dizziness, light-headedness, drowsiness, blurred vision, stomach problems

Drug Interactions

Lorazepam can adversely interact with the following frequently prescribed medications:

- cimetidine (Tagamet)—can cause high lorazepam levels
- disulfiram (Antabuse)—can cause high lorazepam levels
- birth control pills—can cause high lorazepam levels
- alcohol and other drugs that depress certain functions of the nervous system, when combined with lorazepam, can cause extreme drowsiness and slowed reaction times. Examples of these medicines are antihistamines, narcotics, and barbiturates.
- levodopa—decreased effectiveness of levodopa

MEDICAL CONSIDERATIONS

If you have any of the following medical conditions, make sure your doctor is aware of it.

- liver disease or alcoholism—lorazepam levels may be higher than expected
- kidney disease—lorazepam levels may be higher than expected
- drug dependence or alcohol dependence—dependence on lorazepam may occur
- seizure disorder—stopping lorazepam abruptly may cause seizures
- chronic lung disease—lorazepam may make breathing more difficult

---

Drug Name: LOXAPINE   (LOX-a-peen)

Drug Category: Neuroleptic; Antipsychotic
Requires prescription

Commonly Used Brand-Name Products	
Capsules Loxitane (and generic) 5 mg, 10 mg, 25 mg, 50 mg **Liquid** Loxitane C solution 25 mg/ml	**Injection** Loxitane IM 50 mg/ml

GENERAL INFORMATION

Highly effective in treating psychotic symptoms such as hallucinations and delusions. These symptoms occur in schizophrenia, schizoaffective disorder, bipolar disorder or major depression with psychotic features. Also can be used for the short-term management of aggressive, out-of-control behaviors or feelings of anger and rage, and help with symptoms of anxiety and insomnia.

Before Taking this Medication

Talk to your doctor about the benefits and risks associated with loxapine. Make sure you understand how to take it safely and effectively. You and your family members should be very familiar with the side effects. Make sure your doctor has the following information in detail:

- any allergic or bad reactions you have had to loxapine or any other medication
- all prescription and over-the-counter medicines you are taking
- your complete medical history
- if you are pregnant, could be pregnant, or are planning a pregnancy in the near future, loxapine has not been shown to be absolutely safe.
- if you are breast-feeding, loxapine can pass into breast milk and affect the baby

DOSAGE

Adults and adolescents over 16:

Psychotic symptoms: 25–250 mg daily. There is a wide effective dosage range.

Anxiety and insomnia: 5–10 mg daily, usually at bedtime, but in extreme anxiety can be given during waking hours.

Older adults are more susceptible to side effects and generally require lower dosages.

Children and adolescents under 16: Dosages in this age group have not been established.

DIRECTIONS FOR PROPER USE

- *Take exactly as prescribed. Do not take more or less than prescribed.*
- If you take the solution form, the dose must be mixed in orange or grapefruit juice before being taken.
- If you miss a dose, take it as soon as possible. However, if the missed dose is within 4 hours of your next dose, skip the missed dose and resume with your next scheduled dose.
- If you take the liquid form, use the dropper that comes with the bottle to measure out the dose.
- It may take several weeks before you feel the full benefits.

PRECAUTIONS

Alcohol should be avoided while taking loxapine.

Side Effects

Not all side effects will occur. Many side effects will diminish with time. *However, some side effects may be warning signs of toxicity and will require attention from your doctor.* Check with your doctor immediately if you experience any of the following:

- seizure, high fever, fast or irregular heartbeat, very low blood pressure, faintness, any abnormal movements of the mouth, tongue, neck, arms or legs, difficulty speaking or swallowing, imbalance or difficulty walking normally, severe muscle stiffness, discoloration of the skin or eyes, confusion, significant drowsiness, restlessness, difficulty urinating, sexual problems, vomiting, diarrhea, unusual bruising or bleeding, severe skin reaction to sunlight (burning or blistering), severe constipation, breast pain or enlargement

Some side effects appear when you first start taking loxapine and go away for most people. If the following side effects continue, contact your doctor.

- dry mouth, mild to moderate constipation, dizziness, hand tremor, stuffy nose, weight gain

Drug Interactions

Loxapine can adversely interact with the following frequently prescribed medications:

- lithium—increased neurologic side effects
- levodopa—decreased effectiveness of levodopa
- amphetamines—increased psychotic symptoms are possible
- anticonvulsants—decreased loxapine levels
- tricyclic antidepressants—increased TCA levels

MEDICAL CONSIDERATIONS

If you have any of the following medical conditions, make sure your doctor is aware of it.

- kidney disease—loxapine levels may be higher than expected
- liver disease—loxapine levels may be higher than expected
- heart problems—some heart problems can be worsened by loxapine
- seizure disorder—loxapine can lower seizure threshold
- urinary retention, prostate enlargement—urination may be more difficult
- glaucoma—loxapine can increase pressure inside the eye
- Parkinson's disease—some Parkinson's symptoms may be worsened
- breast cancer—may increase risk of cancer progression

Drug Name: MAPROTILINE   (ma-PROE-ti-leen)

Drug Category: Antidepressant, tetracyclic
Requires prescription

Commonly Used Brand-Name Products
Tablets Ludiomil (and generic) 25 mg, 50 mg, 75 mg

GENERAL INFORMATION
Highly effective in treating major depression and the depressed phase of bipolar disorder.

Before Taking this Medication
Talk to your doctor about the benefits and risks associated with maprotiline. Make sure you understand how to take it safely and effectively. Make sure your doctor has the following information in detail:

- any allergic or bad reactions you have had to maprotiline or any other medication
- all prescription and over-the-counter medicines you are taking
- your complete medical history
- if you are pregnant, could be pregnant, or are planning a pregnancy in the near future, maprotiline has not been shown to be absolutely safe
- if you are breast-feeding, maprotiline can pass into breast milk and affect the baby

DOSAGE
The starting dose of maprotiline will be low and gradually be increased.

Adults: Starting dose 25–50 mg at bedtime. Increased to 150–225 mg at bedtime over 2 to 3 weeks.

Children under 18: Safe use and dosages in this age group have not been established.

Older adults are more susceptible to side effects and generally require lower dosages.

DIRECTIONS FOR PROPER USE
- *Take exactly as prescribed. Do not take more or less than prescribed. Accidental or intended overdoses of maprotiline are potentially fatal.*
- If you miss a bedtime dose, do not take it the next morning. It may make you drowsy. Do not double doses.
- It may take several weeks before you feel the full benefits.

- Do not abruptly stop taking maprotiline unless instructed to do so by your doctor. Gradually reducing the dose can help prevent mood changes, headache, or diarrhea.

PRECAUTIONS

Alcohol can cause changes in mood and may interfere with maprotiline's effectiveness. *Alcohol should be avoided while taking maprotiline.*

Side Effects

Not all side effects will occur. Many side effects will diminish with time. *However, some side effects may require attention from your doctor.* Check with your doctor immediately if you experience any of the following:

- seizure, changes in blood pressure, irregular heart rate, shortness of breath, problems with urination, (difficult or painful urination; unable to urinate), confusion, extreme sedation, excitation or mania, increased skin sensitivity to the sunlight, extreme constipation, yellow skin or eyes

Some side effects appear when you first start taking maprotiline and go away for most people. If the following side effects continue, contact your doctor.

- dizziness, blurred vision, dry mouth, mild to moderate constipation, increased appetite, weight gain, breast enlargement (men or women), discharge from the breast, sexual problems, hand tremor, persistent sore throat

Drug Interactions

Maprotiline can adversely interact with the following frequently prescribed medications:

- cimetidine (Tagamet)—can cause high maprotiline levels
- SSRI antidepressants—can cause high maprotiline levels
- MAOI antidepressants—severe reaction causing dangerously high blood pressure, high body temperature, seizures, or death
- clonidine—if clonidine is being taken for high blood pressure, maprotiline may cause it to work less well
- antipsychotics—may increase certain neurologic side effects
- thyroid hormones—increased effects of both, especially excitation and changes in heart rate or rhythm
- drugs used during surgery—can cause increased blood pressure. Make sure your doctors are aware of upcoming planned surgeries

MEDICAL CONSIDERATIONS

If you have any of the following medical conditions, make sure your doctor is aware of it.

- liver disease or alcoholism—maprotiline levels may be higher than expected
- kidney disease—maprotiline levels may be higher than expected
- glaucoma—maprotiline can increase pressure inside the eye
- heart problems—some heart problems can be worsened by maprotiline. It should not be taken by someone who has had a recent heart attack
- urinary retention, prostate enlargement—urination may become more difficult
- seizure disorder—maprotiline can lower seizure threshold
- diabetes mellitus (sugar diabetes)—blood sugar levels may be affected
- thyroid disorders—maprotiline may cause increased heart rate

---

Drug Name: MESORIDAZINE   (meez-o-RID-a-zeen))

Drug Category: Neuroleptic; Antipsychotic
Requires prescription

Commonly Used Brand-Name Products	
Tablets Serentil 10 mg, 25 mg, 50 mg, 100 mg **Liquid** Serentil 25 mg/ml	**Injection** Serentil 25 mg/ml

GENERAL INFORMATION

Highly effective in treating psychotic symptoms, such as hallucinations and delusions. These symptoms occur in schizophrenia, schizoaffective disorder, bipolar disorder or major depression with psychotic features. Also can be used for the short-term management of aggressive, out-of-control behaviors or feelings of anger and rage, and to help with symptoms of anxiety and insomnia.

Before Taking this Medication

Talk to your doctor about the benefits and risks associated with mesoridazine. Make sure you understand how to take it safely and effectively. You and your family members should be very familiar with the side effects. Make sure your doctor has the following information in detail:

- any allergic or bad reactions you have had to mesoridazine or any other medication
- all prescription and over-the-counter medicines you are taking
- your complete medical history
- if you are pregnant, could be pregnant, or are planning a pregnancy in the near future, mesoridazine has not been shown to be absolutely safe
- if you are breast-feeding, mesoridazine can pass into breast milk and affect the baby

DOSAGE

<u>Adults and adolescents over 12:</u>
   <u>Psychotic symptoms:</u> 50–400 mg daily. There is a wide effective dosage range.
   <u>Anxiety and insomnia:</u> 10–25 mg daily, usually at bedtime, but in extreme anxiety can be given during waking hours.
<u>Older adults</u> are more susceptible to side effects and generally require lower dosages.
<u>Children and adolescents under 12:</u> Dosages in this age group have not been established.

DIRECTIONS FOR PROPER USE

- *Take exactly as prescribed. Do not take more or less than prescribed.*
- If you take the solution form, the dose must be mixed in water, or orange or grapefruit juice before being taken.
- If you miss a dose, take it as soon as possible. However, if the missed dose is within 4 hours of your next dose, skip the missed dose and resume with your next scheduled dose.
- If you take the liquid form, avoid contact of the skin with medicine. Irritation can result by the medicine coming into contact with skin. Do not use the liquid form if it becomes discolored or has a sediment at the bottom of the bottle.
- It may take several weeks before you feel the full benefits.

PRECAUTIONS

Alcohol should be avoided while taking mesoridazine.

Side Effects

Not all side effects will occur. Many side effects will diminish with time. *However, some side effects may be warning signs of toxicity and will require attention from your doctor.* Check with your doctor immediately if you experience any of the following:

- seizure, high fever, fast or irregular heartbeat, very low blood pressure, faintness, any abnormal movements of the mouth, tongue, neck, arms or legs, difficulty speaking or swallowing, imbalance or difficulty walking normally, severe muscle stiffness, discoloration of the skin or eyes, confusion, significant drowsiness, restlessness, difficulty urinating, sexual problems, vomiting, diarrhea, unusual bruising or bleeding, severe skin reaction to sunlight (burning or blistering), severe constipation, breast pain or enlargement

Some side effects appear when you first start taking mesoridazine and go away for most people. If the following side effects continue, contact your doctor.

- dry mouth, mild to moderate constipation, dizziness, hand tremor, stuffy nose, weight gain

Drug Interactions

Mesoridazine can adversely interact with the following frequently prescribed medications:

- lithium—increased neurologic side effects
- levodopa—decreased effectiveness of levodopa
- amphetamines—increased psychotic symptoms are possible
- anticonvulsants—decreased mesoridazine levels
- tricyclic antidepressants—increased TCA levels

MEDICAL CONSIDERATIONS

If you have any of the following medical conditions, make sure your doctor is aware of it.

- kidney disease—mesoridazine levels may be higher than expected
- liver disease—mesoridazine levels may be higher than expected
- heart problems—some heart problems can be worsened by mesoridazine
- seizure disorder—mesoridazine can lower seizure threshold
- urinary retention, prostate enlargement—urination may be more difficult
- glaucoma—mesoridazine can increase pressure inside the eye

- Parkinson's disease—some Parkinson's symptoms may be worsened
- breast cancer—may increase risk of cancer progression

Drug Name: METHYLPHENIDATE   (meth-il-FEN-a-date)

Drug Category: Stimulant

Controlled substance, high potential for abuse: Requires special prescription (triplicate, nonrefillable)

Commonly Used Brand-Name Products
Tablets
Ritalin (and generic) 5 mg, 10 mg and 20 mg
Tablets, sustained released
Ritalin SR (and generic) 10 mg and 20 mg

GENERAL INFORMATION

Highly effective in treating Attention Deficit Disorder. Also used to treat narcolepsy (uncontrolled need for sleep or suddenly falling into deep sleep). Can be used to treat major depression.

Before Taking this Medication

Talk to your doctor about the benefits and risks associated with methylphenidate. Make sure you understand how to take it safely and effectively. Make sure your doctor has the following information in detail:

- any allergic or bad reactions you have had to methylphenidate or any other medication
- all prescription and over-the-counter medicines you are taking
- your complete medical history
- if you are pregnant, could be pregnant, or are planning a pregnancy in the near future, methylphenidate has not been shown to be absolutely safe
- if you are breast-feeding, methylphenidate can pass into breast milk and affect the baby

DOSAGE

The starting dose of methylphenidate will be low and gradually be increased.

<u>Adults and children over 6:</u> 5 mg to 20 mg 2 to 3 times daily.

<u>Older adults</u> are more susceptible to side effects and generally require lower dosages.

DIRECTIONS FOR PROPER USE

- *Take exactly as prescribed. Do not take more or less than prescribed. Accidental or intended overdose of methylphenidate is very serious.*
- This medication may work better if taken 30 to 45 minutes before meals.
- If you miss a dose of the regular tablets, take it as soon as possible, unless it is within 3 hours of your next scheduled dose, then skip the missed dose and resume with your next scheduled dose. If you miss a dose of the long-acting tablets, skip the dose and resume with your next scheduled dose. Do not double doses.
- To prevent trouble sleeping at night do not take the last dose later than 6 pm for regular tablets and 3 pm for long-acting tablets, unless otherwise directed by your doctor.
- If you are taking the long-acting form, the tablets should be swallowed whole. Do not crush, break, or chew them.
- Do not abruptly stop taking methylphenidate unless instructed to do so by your doctor.

PRECAUTIONS

Methylphenidate can mask some of the effects of alcohol. Routine alcohol use, or alcohol withdrawal, can increase the chance of seizures, as can methylphenidate. *Alcohol should be avoided while taking methylphenidate.*

Side Effects

Not all side effects will occur. Many side effects will diminish with time. *However, some side effects may require attention from your doctor.* Check with your doctor immediately if you experience any of the following:

- seizure, increased blood pressure, fast or irregular heart rate, shortness of breath, confusion, excitation or mania, severe headache, muscle twitching, unusual behavior, depressed mood, rash or itching

Some side effects appear when you first start taking methylphenidate and go away for most people. If the following side effects continue, contact your doctor.

- dizziness, nervousness, blurred vision, difficulty sleeping, decreased appetite, weight loss

Drug Interactions

Methylphenidate can adversely interact with the following frequently prescribed medications:

- MAOI antidepressants—severe reaction causing dangerously high blood pressure, high body temperature, seizures, or death
- other stimulant medicines—decongestants, diet pills, some asthma medications, caffeine
- pimozide—methylphenidate may worsen tics

MEDICAL CONSIDERATIONS

If you have any of the following medical conditions, make sure your doctor is aware of it.

- liver disease or alcoholism—methylphenidate levels may be higher than expected
- seizure disorder—methylphenidate may increase the chance of seizures
- kidney disease—methylphenidate levels may be higher than expected
- alcohol or drug abuse—dependence on methylphenidate may result
- heart problems—some heart problems can be worsened by methylphenidate
- glaucoma—methylphenidate may raise intraocular pressure
- high blood pressure—methylphenidate may increase blood pressure
- Tourette's syndrome—methylphenidate may worsen tics

Drug Name: MIRTAZAPINE   (mur-TAZ-a-peen)

Drug Category: Antidepressant, atypical
Requires prescription

Commonly Used Brand-Name Products
Tablets Remeron 15 mg, 30 mg

GENERAL INFORMATION

Effective in treating major depression.

Before Taking this Medication

Talk to your doctor about the benefits and risks associated with mirtazapine. Make sure you understand how to take it safely and effectively. Make sure your doctor has the following information in detail:

- any allergic or bad reactions you have had to mirtazapine or any other medication
- all prescription and over-the-counter medicines you are taking
- your complete medical history
- if you are pregnant, could be pregnant, or are planning a pregnancy in the near future, mirtazapine has not been shown to be absolutely safe
- if you are breast-feeding, mirtazapine can pass into breast milk and affect the baby

DOSAGE

The starting dose of mirtazapine will be low and gradually be increased depending on your response and the side effects.

<u>Adults:</u> 15–45 mg daily, usually at bedtime.

<u>Older adults</u> are more susceptible to side effects and generally require lower dosages.

<u>Children and adolescents under 18:</u> Safe use and dosages in this age group have not been established.

DIRECTIONS FOR PROPER USE

- *Take exactly as prescribed. Do not take more or less than prescribed.*
- If you miss a dose, skip the missed dose and resume with your next scheduled dose. Do not double doses.
- It may take several weeks before you feel the full benefits.
- Do not abruptly stop taking mirtazapine unless instructed to do so by your doctor.

PRECAUTIONS

Alcohol can cause changes in mood and may interfere with mirtazapine's effectiveness. *Alcohol should be avoided while taking mirtazapine.*

Side Effects

Not all side effects will occur. Many side effects will diminish with time. *However, some side effects may require attention from your doctor.* Check with your doctor immediately if you experience any of the following:

- extreme drowsiness, decreased blood pressure, decreased heart rate, skin rash or hives, shortness of breath, chills or fever, swelling of the hands or feet, seizures

Some side effects appear when you first start taking mirtazapine and go away for most people. If the following side effects continue, contact your doctor.

- dizziness, increased appetite, weight gain, dry mouth, constipation

Drug Interactions

Mirtazapine can adversely interact with the following frequently prescribed medications:

- anticoagulants (blood thinners)—the effect of the anticoagulant can be increased
- some nonsedating antihistamines—cardiac (heart) toxicity
- diet pills—severe reaction causing dangerously high blood pressure, high body temperature, seizures, or death
- products containing l-tryptophan—severe reaction causing dangerously high blood pressure, high body temperature, seizures, or death
- cimetidine (Tagamet)—can cause high mirtazapine levels
- TCA antidepressants—can cause high TCA levels
- MAOI antidepressants—severe reaction causing dangerously high blood pressure, high body temperature, seizures, or death
- antipsychotics—may increase certain neurologic side effects
- lithium—increased lithium levels may cause confusion, dizziness, tremor
- anticonvulsants—increased anticonvulsant levels or decreased mirtazapine levels

MEDICAL CONSIDERATIONS

If you have any of the following medical conditions, make sure your doctor is aware of it.

- liver disease or alcoholism—mirtazapine levels may be higher than expected
- kidney disease—mirtazapine levels may be higher than expected
- seizure disorder—mirtazapine can lower seizure threshold
- diabetes mellitus (sugar diabetes)—blood sugar levels may be affected

Drug Name: MOLINDONE   (moe-LIN-doan)

Drug Category: Neuroleptic; Antipsychotic
Requires prescription

Commonly Used Brand-Name Products
Tablets Moban 5 mg, 10 mg, 25 mg, 50 mg, 100 mg **Liquid** Moban 20 mg/ml

GENERAL INFORMATION
Highly effective in treating psychotic symptoms, such as halluci-nations and delusions. These symptoms occur in schizophrenia, schizoaffective disorder, bipolar disorder or major depression with psychotic features.

Before Taking this Medication
Talk to your doctor about the benefits and risks associated with molindone. Make sure you understand how to take it safely and effectively. You and your family members should be very familiar with the side effects. Make sure your doctor has the following in-formation in detail:

- any allergic or bad reactions you have had to molindone or any other medication
- all prescription and over-the-counter medicines you are taking
- your complete medical history
- if you are pregnant, could be pregnant, or are planning a preg-nancy in the near future, molindone has not been shown to be absolutely safe
- if you are breast-feeding, molindone can pass into breast milk and affect the baby.

DOSAGE
Adults and adolescents over 12:
  Psychotic symptoms: 50–225 mg daily. There is a wide effective
  dosage range.
Older adults are more susceptible to side effects and generally re-quire lower dosages.
Children and adolescents under 12: Dosages in this age group have not been established.

DIRECTIONS FOR PROPER USE

- *Take exactly as prescribed. Do not take more or less than pre- scribed.*
- If you take the solution form, it may be mixed in milk, water, orange or grapefruit juice before taking.
- If you miss a dose, take it as soon as possible. However, if the missed dose is within 4 hours of your next dose, skip the missed dose and resume with your next scheduled dose.
- If you take the liquid form, avoid contact of the skin with medi- cine. Irritation can result by the medicine coming into contact with skin. Do not use the liquid form if it becomes discolored or has a sediment at the bottom of the bottle.
- It may take several weeks before you feel the full benefits.

PRECAUTIONS

Alcohol should be avoided while taking molindone.

Side Effects

Not all side effects will occur. Many side effects will diminish with time. *However, some side effects may be warning signs of toxicity and will require attention from your doctor.* Check with your doctor immediately if you experience any of the following:

- seizure, high fever, fast or irregular heartbeat, very low blood pressure, faintness, any abnormal movements of the mouth, tongue, neck, arms or legs, difficulty speaking or swallowing, imbalance or difficulty walking normally, severe muscle stiff- ness, discoloration of the skin or eyes, confusion, significant drowsiness, restlessness, difficulty urinating, sexual problems, vomiting, diarrhea, unusual bruising or bleeding, severe skin reaction to sunlight (burning or blistering), severe constipation, breast pain or enlargement

Some side effects appear when you first start taking molindone and go away for most people. If the following side effects con- tinue, contact your doctor.

- dry mouth, mild to moderate constipation, dizziness, hand tremor, stuffy nose, weight gain

Drug Interactions

Molindone can adversely interact with the following frequently prescribed medications:

- lithium—increased neurologic side effects
- levodopa—decreased effectiveness of levodopa
- amphetamines—increased psychotic symptoms are possible

- anticonvulsants—decreased molindone levels
- tricyclic antidepressants—increased TCA levels

MEDICAL CONSIDERATIONS

If you have any of the following medical conditions, make sure your doctor is aware of it.

- kidney disease—molindone levels may be higher than expected
- liver disease—molindone levels may be higher than expected
- heart problems—some heart problems can be worsened by molindone
- seizure disorder—molindone can lower seizure threshold
- urinary retention, prostate enlargement—urination may be more difficult
- glaucoma—molindone can increase pressure inside the eye
- Parkinson's disease—some Parkinson's symptoms may be worsened
- breast cancer—may increase risk of cancer progression

Drug Name: NEFAZODONE   (ne-FAZ-oh-doan)

Drug Category: Antidepressant, atypical
Requires prescription

Commonly Used Brand-Name Products
Tablets
Serzone 100 mg, 150 mg, 200 mg, 250 mg

GENERAL INFORMATION

Highly effective in treating major depression and the depressed phase of bipolar disorder.

Before Taking this Medication

Talk to your doctor about the benefits and risks associated with nefazodone. Make sure you understand how to take it safely and effectively. Make sure your doctor has the following information in detail:

- any allergic or bad reactions you have had to nefazodone or any other medication
- all prescription and over-the-counter medicines you are taking
- your complete medical history

- if you are pregnant, could be pregnant, or are planning a pregnancy in the near future, nefazodone has not been shown to be absolutely safe
- if you are breast-feeding, nefazodone can pass into breast milk and affect the baby

DOSAGE

The starting dose of nefazodone will be low and gradually be increased.

Adults: Starting dose 100 mg 2 times daily. Increased to 200–600 mg at bedtime over 2 to 3 weeks.

Older adults are more susceptible to side effects and generally require lower dosages.

Children and adolescents under 18: Safe use and dosages in this age group have not been established.

DIRECTIONS FOR PROPER USE

- *Take exactly as prescribed. Do not take more or less than prescribed. Accidental or intended overdoses of nefazodone are potentially fatal.*
- Take with food or milk to lessen stomach upset.
- If you miss a dose, take it as soon as possible, unless it is within 6 hours of your next scheduled dose, then skip the missed dose and resume with your next scheduled dose. Do not double doses.
- It may take several weeks before you feel the full benefits.
- Do not abruptly stop taking nefazodone unless instructed to do so by your doctor. Gradually reducing the dose can help prevent mood changes, headache, or diarrhea.

PRECAUTIONS

Alcohol can cause changes in mood and may interfere with nefazodone's effectiveness. *Alcohol should be avoided while taking nefazodone.*

Side Effects

Not all side effects will occur. Many side effects will diminish with time. *However, some side effects may require attention from your doctor.* Check with your doctor immediately if you experience any of the following:

- seizure, changes in blood pressure, irregular heart rate, shortness of breath, problems with urination, (difficult or painful urination; unable to urinate), confusion, extreme sedation, excitation or mania, increased skin sensitivity to sunlight, extreme constipation, yellow skin or eyes

Some side effects appear when you first start taking nefazodone and go away for most people. If the following side effects continue, contact your doctor.

- dizziness, blurred vision, dry mouth, mild to moderate constipation, increased appetite, weight gain, breast enlargement (men or women), discharge from the breast, sexual problems, hand tremor, persistent sore throat

Drug Interactions

Nefazodone can adversely interact with the following frequently prescribed medications:

- SSRI antidepressants—can cause high nefazodone levels
- MAOI antidepressants—severe reaction causing dangerously high blood pressure, high body temperature, seizures, or death
- some nonsedating antihistamines—cardiac (heart) toxicity
- clonidine—if clonidine is being taken for high blood pressure, nefazodone may cause it to work less well
- antipsychotics—may increase certain neurologic side effects
- drugs used during surgery—can cause increased blood pressure. Make sure your doctors are aware of upcoming planned surgeries

MEDICAL CONSIDERATIONS

If you have any of the following medical conditions, make sure your doctor is aware of it. Nefazodone may affect your condition.

- liver disease or alcoholism—nefazodone levels may be higher than expected
- kidney disease—nefazodone levels may be higher than expected
- heart problems—some heart problems can be worsened by nefazodone. Nefazodone should not be taken by someone who has had a recent heart attack
- urinary retention, prostate enlargement—urination may become more difficult

---

Drug Name: NORTRIPTYLINE   (nor-TRIP-ti-leen)

Drug Category: Antidepressant, tricyclic
Requires prescription

Commonly Used Brand-Name Products
Capsules Pamelor, Aventyl (and generic) 10 mg, 25 mg, 50 mg, 75 mg **Solution** Pamelor, Aventyl (and generic) 10 mg/tsp (contains alcohol)

GENERAL INFORMATION

Highly effective in treating major depression and the depressed phase of bipolar disorder. Effective in treating panic disorder. Due to its sedative effects, it is sometimes given in low doses to help with insomnia. Also used to treat certain chronic pain disorders, such as migraine headache and diabetic neuropathy.

Before Taking this Medication

Talk to your doctor about the benefits and risks associated with nortriptyline. Make sure you understand how to take it safely and effectively. Make sure your doctor has the following information in detail:

- any allergic or bad reactions you have had to nortriptyline or any other medication
- all prescription and over-the-counter medicines you are taking
- your complete medical history
- if you are pregnant, could be pregnant, or are planning a pregnancy in the near future, nortriptyline has not been shown to be absolutely safe
- if you are breast-feeding, nortriptyline can pass into breast milk and affect the baby

DOSAGE

The starting dose of nortriptyline will be low and gradually be increased.

Adults:

Depression: Starting dose 10–25 mg at bedtime. Increased to 75–150 mg at bedtime over 2 to 3 weeks.

Insomnia: 10–25 mg at bedtime.

Chronic pain syndromes: 10–50 mg daily.

Adolescents: Adolescents may be more susceptible to heart-related side effects. Blood levels and heart function should be monitored.

Children 6–12: Safe use and dosages in this age group have not been established. When used in children, dose is based on body weight. Children are more susceptible to serious heart-related side effects. Blood levels and heart function should be monitored.

<u>Older adults</u> are more susceptible to side effects and generally require lower dosages.

DIRECTIONS FOR PROPER USE

- *Take exactly as prescribed. Do not take more or less than prescribed. Accidental or intended overdoses of nortriptyline are potentially fatal.*
- If you miss a bedtime dose, do not take it the next morning. It may make you drowsy. Do not double doses.
- It may take several weeks before you feel the full benefits.
- Laboratory tests may be done to determine if the amount of nortriptyline in your bloodstream is in the correct range.
- Do not abruptly stop taking nortriptyline unless instructed to do so by your doctor. Gradually reducing the dose can help prevent mood changes, headache, or diarrhea.

PRECAUTIONS

Alcohol can cause changes in mood and may interfere with nortriptyline's effectiveness. *Alcohol should be avoided while taking nortriptyline.*

Side Effects

Not all side effects will occur. Many side effects will diminish with time. *However, some side effects may require attention from your doctor.* Check with your doctor immediately if you experience any of the following:

- seizure, changes in blood pressure, irregular heart rate, shortness of breath, problems with urination, (difficult or painful urination; unable to urinate), confusion, extreme sedation, excitation or mania, increased skin sensitivity to sunlight, extreme constipation, yellow skin or eyes

Some side effects appear when you first start taking nortriptyline and go away for most people. If the following side effects continue, contact your doctor.

- dizziness, blurred vision, dry mouth, mild to moderate constipation, increased appetite, weight gain, breast enlargement (men or women), discharge from the breast, sexual problems, hand tremor, persistent sore throat

Drug Interactions

Nortriptyline can adversely interact with the following frequently prescribed medications:

- cimetidine (Tagamet)—can cause high nortriptyline levels

- SSRI antidepressants—can cause high nortriptyline levels
- MAOI antidepressants—severe reaction causing dangerously high blood pressure, high body temperature, seizures, or death
- clonidine—if clonidine is being taken for high blood pressure, nortriptyline may cause it to work less well
- antipsychotics—may increase certain neurologic side effects
- thyroid hormones—increased effects of both, especially excitation and changes in heart rate or rhythm
- drugs used during surgery—can cause increased blood pressure. Make sure your doctors are aware of upcoming planned surgeries

MEDICAL CONSIDERATIONS

If you have any of the following medical conditions, make sure your doctor is aware of it.

- liver disease or alcoholism—nortriptyline levels may be higher than expected
- kidney disease—nortriptyline levels may be higher than expected
- glaucoma—nortriptyline can increase pressure inside the eye
- heart problems—some heart problems can be worsened by nortriptyline. Nortriptyline should not be taken by someone who has had a recent heart attack
- urinary retention, prostate enlargement—urination may become more difficult
- seizure disorder—nortriptyline can lower seizure threshold
- diabetes mellitus (sugar diabetes)—blood sugar levels may be affected
- thyroid disorders—nortriptyline may cause increased heart rate

---

Drug Name: OLANZAPINE   (o-LANZ-a-peen)

Drug Category: Neuroleptic; Antipsychotic
Requires prescription

Commonly Used Brand-Name Products
Tablets
Zyprexa 5 mg, 10 mg

GENERAL INFORMATION

Highly effective in treating psychotic symptoms, such as hallucinations and delusions. Olanzapine has been most widely studied in schizophrenia, but may also be useful in treating the psychotic symptoms associated with schizoaffective disorder, bipolar disorder, or major depression with psychotic features.

Before Taking this Medication

Talk to your doctor about the benefits and risks associated with olanzapine. Make sure you understand how to take it safely and effectively. You and your family members should be very familiar with the side effects. Make sure your doctor has the following information in detail:

- any allergic or bad reactions you have had to olanzapine or any other medication
- all prescription and over-the-counter medicines you are taking
- your complete medical history
- if you are pregnant, could be pregnant, or are planning a pregnancy in the near future, olanzapine has not been shown to be absolutely safe
- if you are breast-feeding, olanzapine can pass into breast milk and affect the baby

DOSAGE

Adults:

   Psychotic symptoms: 5–20 mg daily.

Older adults are more susceptible to side effects and generally require lower dosages.

Children: Dosages in this age group have not been established.

DIRECTIONS FOR PROPER USE

- *Take exactly as prescribed. Do not take more or less than prescribed.*
- If you miss a dose, take it as soon as possible. However, if the missed dose is within 4 hours of your next dose, skip the missed dose and resume with your next scheduled dose.
- It may take several weeks before you feel the full benefits.

PRECAUTIONS

Alcohol should be avoided while taking olanzapine.

Side Effects

Not all side effects will occur. Many side effects will diminish with time. *However, some side effects may be warning signs of toxicity and will require attention from your doctor.* Check with your doctor immediately if you experience any of the following:

- seizure, high fever, fast or irregular heartbeat, very low blood pressure, faintness, any abnormal movements of the mouth, tongue, neck, arms or legs, difficulty speaking or swallowing, imbalance or difficulty walking normally, severe muscle stiffness, discoloration of the skin or eyes, confusion, significant drowsiness, restlessness, difficulty urinating, sexual problems, vomiting, diarrhea, unusual bruising or bleeding, severe skin reaction to sunlight (burning or blistering), severe constipation, breast pain or enlargement

Some side effects appear when you first start taking olanzapine and go away for most people. If the following side effects continue, contact your doctor.

- dry mouth, nausea, vomiting, mild to moderate constipation, dizziness, hand tremor, stuffy nose, weight gain

Drug Interactions
Olanzapine can adversely interact with the following frequently prescribed medications:

- lithium—increased neurologic side effects
- levodopa—decreased effectiveness of levodopa
- amphetamines—increased psychotic symptoms are possible
- anticonvulsants—decreased olanzapine levels
- tricyclic antidepressants—increased TCA levels

MEDICAL CONSIDERATIONS
If you have any of the following medical conditions, make sure your doctor is aware of it.

- kidney disease—olanzapine levels may be higher than expected
- liver disease—olanzapine levels may be higher than expected
- heart problems—some heart problems can be worsened by olanzapine
- seizure disorder—olanzapine can lower seizure threshold
- urinary retention, prostate enlargement—urination may be more difficult
- glaucoma—olanzapine can increase pressure inside the eye
- Parkinson's disease—some Parkinson's symptoms may be worsened
- breast cancer—may increase risk of cancer progression

Drug Name: OXAZEPAM   (ox-AZ-e-pam)

Drug Category: Antianxiety medicine

Requires prescription, controlled substance, moderate potential for abuse

Commonly Used Brand-Name Products
Capsules
Serax (and generic) 10mg, 15mg, 30mg
Tablets
Serax (and generic) 10mg, 15mg, 30mg

GENERAL INFORMATION

Highly effective in treating anxiety and nervousness, also used to treat symptoms of alcohol withdrawal.

Before Taking this Medication

Talk to your doctor about the benefits and risks associated with oxazepam. Make sure you understand how to take it safely and effectively. You and your family members should be very familiar with the side effects and signs of having too much oxazepam in your system. Make sure your doctor has the following information in detail:

- any allergic or bad reactions you have had to oxazepam or any other medication
- all prescription and over-the-counter medicines you are taking
- your complete medical history
- if you are pregnant, could be pregnant, or are planning a pregnancy in the near future, oxazepam should not be taken
- if you are breast-feeding, oxazepam can pass into breast milk and affect the baby

DOSAGE

Adults: 10-30 mg 2 to 3 times a day.

Older adults are more susceptible to side effects and generally require lower dosages.

Children under 12: When used in children, dosage is based on body weight.

DIRECTIONS FOR PROPER USE

- *Take exactly as prescribed. Do not take more or less than pre-scribed. Oxazepam levels that are too high can cause serious toxicity.*
- Take with food if stomach upset occurs.
- If you take oxazepam regularly for an extended period of time, do not stop taking it unless told to do so by your doctor. It may be necessary to gradually reduce the dose before stopping completely.
- If you miss a dose, take it as soon as possible. However, if the missed dose is within 4 hours of your next dose, skip the missed dose and resume with your next scheduled dose.

PRECAUTIONS

Alcohol should be avoided while taking oxazepam.

Side Effects

Not all side effects will occur. Many side effects will diminish with time. *However, some side effects may be warning signs of toxicity and will require attention from your doctor.* Check with your doctor immediately if you experience any of the following:

- confusion, severe drowsiness, slurred speech, severe weakness, unusual thoughts, shortness of breath, excitement, hyperactivity

Some side effects appear when you first start taking oxazepam and go away for most people. If the following side effects continue, contact your doctor.

- dizziness, light-headedness, drowsiness, blurred vision, stomach problems

Drug Interactions

Oxazepam can adversely interact with the following frequently prescribed medications:

- cimetidine (Tagamet)—can cause high oxazepam levels
- disulfiram (Antabuse)—can cause high oxazepam levels
- birth control pills—can cause high oxazepam levels
- alcohol and other drugs that depress certain functions of the nervous system, when combined with oxazepam, can cause extreme drowsiness and slowed reaction times. Examples of these medicines are antihistamines, narcotics, and barbiturates
- levodopa—decreased effectiveness of levodopa

MEDICAL CONSIDERATIONS

If you have any of the following medical conditions, make sure your doctor is aware of it.

- liver disease or alcoholism—oxazepam levels may be higher than expected
- kidney disease—oxazepam levels may be higher than expected
- drug dependence or alcohol dependence—dependence on oxazepam may occur
- seizure disorder—stopping oxazepam abruptly may cause seizures
- chronic lung disease—oxazepam may make breathing more difficult

---

Drug Name: PAROXETINE   (pa-ROX-a-teen)

Drug Category: Antidepressant, SSRI
(serotonin specific reuptake inhibitor)
Requires prescription

Commonly Used Brand-Name Products
Tablets Paxil 10 mg, 20 mg, 30 mg, 40 mg

GENERAL INFORMATION

Highly effective in treating major depression and the depressed phase of bipolar disorder. May be effective in treating obsessive compulsive disorder (OCD), panic disorder, and bulimia. Also may be used to treat attention deficit hyperactivity disorder, especially in adults.

Before Taking this Medication

Talk to your doctor about the benefits and risks associated with paroxetine. Make sure you understand how to take it safely and effectively. Make sure your doctor has the following information in detail:

- any allergic or bad reactions you have had to paroxetine or any other medication
- all prescription and over-the-counter medicines you are taking
- your complete medical history

- if you are pregnant, could be pregnant, or are planning a pregnancy in the near future, paroxetine has not been shown to be absolutely safe
- if you are breast-feeding, paroxetine can pass into breast milk and affect the baby

DOSAGE
Adults:
   Depression, panic disorder, bulimia: 10–40 mg daily. Sometimes higher doses are required. Dosage increases should not be more often than every 1 to 2 weeks.
   OCD: 20–50 mg daily.
Children and adolescents: Safe use has not been established.
Older adults are more susceptible to side effects and generally require lower dosages.

DIRECTIONS FOR PROPER USE
- *Take exactly as prescribed. Do not take more or less than prescribed.*
- May be taken with food or meals to lessen stomach upset.
- If you miss a dose, do not try to make it up. Wait and take your next scheduled dose. Do not double doses.
- It may take several weeks before you feel the full benefits.
- Do not abruptly stop taking paroxetine unless instructed to do so by your doctor.

PRECAUTIONS
Alcohol can cause changes in mood and may interfere with paroxetine's effectiveness. *Alcohol should be avoided while taking paroxetine.*

Side Effects
Not all side effects will occur. Many side effects will diminish with time. *However, some side effects may require attention from your doctor.* Check with your doctor immediately if you experience any of the following:
- skin rash or hives, shortness of breath, chills or fever, swelling of the hands or feet, seizures, sore throat

Some side effects appear when you first start taking paroxetine and go away for most people. If the following side effects continue, contact your doctor.
- stimulation, anxiety, insomnia, dizziness, sexual problems, sweating, blurred vision, dry mouth, mild to moderate constipa-

tion, change in appetite, change in weight, hand tremor, head-ache

Drug Interactions

Paroxetine can adversely interact with the following frequently prescribed medications:

- anticoagulants (blood thinners)—the effect of the anticoagulant can be increased
- some nonsedating antihistamines—cardiac (heart) toxicity
- diet pills—severe reaction causing dangerously high blood pressure, high body temperature, seizures, or death
- cimetidine (Tagamet)—can cause high paroxetine levels
- TCA antidepressants—can cause high TCA levels
- MAOI antidepressants—severe reaction causing dangerously high blood pressure, high body temperature, seizures, or death
- antipsychotics—may increase certain neurologic side effects
- lithium—increased lithium levels may cause confusion, dizziness, tremor
- anticonvulsants—increased anticonvulsant levels or decreased paroxetine levels

MEDICAL CONSIDERATIONS

If you have any of the following medical conditions, make sure your doctor is aware of it.

- liver disease or alcoholism—paroxetine levels may be higher than expected
- kidney disease—paroxetine levels may be higher than expected
- seizure disorder—paroxetine can lower seizure threshold
- diabetes mellitus (sugar diabetes)—blood sugar levels may be affected

---

Drug Name: PEMOLINE   (pem-O-leen)

Drug Category: Stimulant

Requires prescription, controlled substance, low potential for abuse

Commonly Used Brand-Name Products
Tablets Cylert 18.75 mg, 37.5 mg and 75 mg **Tablets, chewable** Cylert 37.5 mg

GENERAL INFORMATION
Highly effective in treating Attention Deficit Disorder. Also used to treat narcolepsy (uncontrolled need for sleep or suddenly falling into deep sleep).

Before Taking this Medication
Talk to your doctor about the benefits and risks associated with pemoline. Make sure you understand how to take it safely and effectively. Make sure your doctor has the following information in detail:

- any allergic or bad reactions you have had to pemoline or any other medication
- all prescription and over-the-counter medicines you are taking
- your complete medical history
- if you are pregnant, could be pregnant, or are planning a pregnancy in the near future, pemoline has not been shown to be absolutely safe
- if you are breast-feeding, pemoline can pass into breast milk and affect the baby

DOSAGE
The starting dose of pemoline will be low and gradually be increased.

Adults and children over 6: 37.5 mg to 112.5 mg daily.

Older adults are more susceptible to side effects and generally require lower dosages.

DIRECTIONS FOR PROPER USE
- *Take exactly as prescribed. Do not take more or less than prescribed. Accidental or intended overdoses of pemoline are very serious.*
- If you miss a dose, take it as soon as possible. Do not double doses.
- The chewable tablets should be thoroughly chewed. Do not swallow whole.

- To prevent difficulty sleeping at night, pemoline should be taken in the morning.
- Do not abruptly stop taking pemoline unless instructed to do so by your doctor.

PRECAUTIONS

Routine alcohol use, or alcohol withdrawal, can increase the chance of seizures, as can pemoline. *Alcohol should be avoided while taking pemoline.*

Side Effects

Not all side effects will occur. Many side effects will diminish with time. *However, some side effects may require attention from your doctor.* Check with your doctor immediately if you experience any of the following:

- seizure, increased blood pressure, fast or irregular heart rate, shortness of breath, confusion, excitation or mania, severe headache, muscle twitching, unusual behavior, depressed mood, rash or itching, yellow skin or eyes

Some side effects appear when you first start taking pemoline and go away for most people. If the following side effects continue, contact your doctor.

- dizziness, nervousness, blurred vision, difficulty sleeping, decreased appetite, weight loss

Drug Interactions

Pemoline can adversely interact with the following frequently prescribed medications:

- MAOI antidepressants—severe reaction causing dangerously high blood pressure, high body temperature, seizures, or death
- other stimulant medicines—decongestants, diet pills, some asthma medications, caffeine
- anticonvulsants—pemoline may increase the chance of seizures, thus requiring an adjustment in the dose of anticonvulsants

MEDICAL CONSIDERATIONS

If you have any of the following medical conditions, make sure your doctor is aware of it.

- liver disease or alcoholism—pemoline levels may be higher than expected. Damage to the liver may be worsened.
- seizure disorder—pemoline may increase the chance of seizures
- kidney disease—pemoline levels may be higher than expected
- alcohol or drug abuse—dependence on pemoline may result
- Tourette's syndrome—pemoline may worsen tics

Drug Name: PERPHENAZINE   (per-FEN-a-zeen)

Drug Category: Neuroleptic; Antipsychotic
Requires prescription

Commonly Used Brand-Name Products	
Tablets Trilafon (and generic), 2 mg, 4 mg, 8 mg, 16 mg **Liquid** Trilafon (and generic) solution 16 mg/5ml (contains alcohol)	**Injection** Trilafon, 5 mg/ml

GENERAL INFORMATION
Highly effective in treating psychotic symptoms, such as hallucinations and delusions. These symptoms occur in schizophrenia, schizoaffective disorder, bipolar disorder, or major depression with psychotic features. Also can be used for the short-term management of aggressive, out-of-control behaviors or feelings of anger and rage, and to help with symptoms of anxiety and insomnia.

Before Taking this Medication
Talk to your doctor about the benefits and risks associated with perphenazine. Make sure you understand how to take it safely and effectively. You and your family members should be very familiar with the side effects. Make sure your doctor has the following information in detail:
- any allergic or bad reactions you have had to perphenazine or any other medication
- all prescription and over-the-counter medicines you are taking
- your complete medical history
- if you are pregnant, could be pregnant, or are planning a pregnancy in the near future, perphenazine has not been shown to be absolutely safe
- if you are breast-feeding, perphenazine can pass into breast milk and affect the baby

DOSAGE
Adults and adolescents:
   Psychotic symptoms: 4–64 mg daily. There is a wide effective dosage range.

Anxiety and insomnia: 2–4 mg daily, usually at bedtime, but in extreme anxiety can be given during waking hours.

Older adults are more susceptible to side effects and generally require lower dosages.

Children under 12: Dosages in this age group have not been established.

DIRECTIONS FOR PROPER USE

- *Take exactly as prescribed. Do not take more or less than prescribed.*
- If you are taking the liquid form it must be diluted before swallowing. It may be diluted in water, milk, tomato or fruit juices, except apple juice. It should not be mixed with coffee, tea, or colas. The dose should be measured carefully.
- If you are taking the solution form, avoid contact of the skin with the medicine. Irritation can result by the medicine coming into contact with skin. Do not use the liquid form if it becomes very discolored (dark yellow) or has a sediment at the bottom of the bottle.
- If you miss a dose, take it as soon as possible. However, if the missed dose is within 4 hours of your next dose, skip the missed dose and resume with your next scheduled dose.
- It may take several weeks before you feel the full benefits.

PRECAUTIONS

Alcohol should be avoided while taking perphenazine.

Side Effects

Not all side effects will occur. Many side effects will diminish with time. *However, some side effects may be warning signs of toxicity and will require attention from your doctor.* Check with your doctor immediately if you experience any of the following:

- seizure, high fever, fast or irregular heartbeat, very low blood pressure, faintness, any abnormal movements of the mouth, tongue, neck, arms or legs, difficulty speaking or swallowing, imbalance or difficulty walking normally, severe muscle stiffness, discoloration of the skin or eyes, confusion, significant drowsiness, restlessness, difficulty urinating, sexual problems, vomiting, diarrhea, unusual bruising or bleeding, severe skin reaction to sunlight (burning or blistering), severe constipation, breast pain or enlargement

Some side effects appear when you first start taking perphenazine and go away for most people. If the following side effects continue, contact your doctor.

- dry mouth, mild to moderate constipation, dizziness, hand tremor, stuffy nose, weight gain

Drug Interactions

Perphenazine can adversely interact with the following frequently prescribed medications:

- lithium—increased neurologic side effects
- levodopa—decreased effectiveness of levodopa
- amphetamines—increased psychotic symptoms are possible
- anticonvulsants—decreased perphenazine levels
- tricyclic antidepressants—increased TCA levels

MEDICAL CONSIDERATIONS

If you have any of the following medical conditions, make sure your doctor is aware of it.

- kidney disease—perphenazine levels may be higher than expected
- liver disease—perphenazine levels may be higher than expected
- heart problems—some heart problems can be worsened by perphenazine
- seizure disorder—perphenazine can lower seizure threshold
- urinary retention, prostate enlargement—urination may be more difficult
- glaucoma—perphenazine can increase pressure inside the eye
- Parkinson's disease—some Parkinson's symptoms may be worsened
- breast cancer—may increase risk of cancer progression

Drug Name: PHENELZINE   (fen-EL-zeen)

Drug Category: Antidepressant, MAOI
(monoamine oxidase inhibitor)
Requires prescription

Commonly Used Brand-Name Products
Tablets Nardil 15 mg

GENERAL INFORMATION

Highly effective in treating major depression, and the depressed phase of bipolar disorder. Also very effective in treating panic disorder, and effective in treating social phobia.

Before Taking this Medication

Talk to your doctor about the benefits and risks associated with phenelzine. Make sure you understand how to take it safely and effectively. Make sure your doctor has the following information in detail:

- any allergic or bad reactions you have had to phenelzine or any other medication
- all prescription and over-the-counter medicines you are taking
- your complete medical history
- if you are pregnant, could be pregnant, or are planning a pregnancy in the near future, phenelzine has not been shown to be absolutely safe
- if you are breast-feeding, phenelzine can pass into breast milk and affect the baby

DOSAGE

The starting dose of phenelzine will be low and gradually be increased.

Adults: 30–60 mg daily.

Older adults are more susceptible to side effects and generally require lower dosages.

Children under 16: Safe use and dosages in this age group have not been established.

DIRECTIONS FOR PROPER USE

- *Take exactly as prescribed. Do not take more or less than prescribed. Accidental or intended overdoses of phenelzine are potentially fatal.*
- *Follow the dietary instructions described below carefully while taking phenelzine. Not doing so can lead to dangerously high blood pressure.*
- The amount of tyramine, or tryptophan, in your diet must be restricted while taking phenelzine. Tyramine is found in foods that have been aged, preserved, or that have undergone protein breakdown. The amount of tyramine in food is **not** inactivated by cooking. These restrictions must be followed for two weeks after phenelzine has been stopped. (See "Foods to Avoid Completely" in chapter 5 on page 63.)

- *Check with your doctor or pharmacist before taking any other prescription or over-the-counter medicine.*
- It is advised that you check your blood pressure frequently while taking phenelzine.
- If you miss a bedtime dose, do not take it the next morning since it may make you drowsy. Do not double doses.
- It may take several weeks before you feel the full benefits.
- Do not abruptly stop taking phenelzine unless instructed to do so by your doctor. Gradually reducing the dose can help prevent mood changes, headache, or diarrhea.

PRECAUTIONS

Alcohol can cause changes in mood and may interfere with phenelzine's effectiveness. *Alcohol should be avoided while taking phenelzine.*

Side Effects

Not all side effects will occur. Many side effects will diminish with time. *However, some side effects may require attention from your doctor.* Check with your doctor immediately if you experience any of the following:

- seizure, changes in blood pressure, severe headache, irregular heart rate, shortness of breath, problems with urination, (difficult or painful urination; unable to urinate), confusion, extreme sedation, excitation or mania, extreme sweating, severe skin sensitivity to sunlight (burning or blistering), extreme constipation, yellow skin or eyes

Some side effects appear when you first start taking phenelzine and go away for most people. If the following side effects continue, contact your doctor.

- dizziness, blurred vision, dry mouth, mild to moderate constipation, increased appetite, weight gain, tremor of the hands

Drug Interactions

Phenelzine can adversely interact with the following frequently prescribed medications. A severe reaction causing dangerously high blood pressure, high body temperature, seizures, or death is possible. These interactions are possible for up to 2 weeks after phenelzine has been stopped. A "washout" period of up to 5 weeks after stopping some of the medications listed below may be necessary before starting phenelzine.

- SSRI antidepressants
- TCA antidepressants

- stimulant drugs—amphetamines, methylphenidate (Ritalin), cocaine
- ephedrine, pseudoephedrine—found in prescription and over-the-counter cough, cold, or asthma medicines
- phenylephrine, phenylpropanolamine—found in prescription and over-the-counter cough, cold, or asthma medicines
- levodopa
- buspirone (Buspar)
- dextromethorphan—found in prescription and over-the-counter cough syrups and lozenges
- meperidine (Demerol)

MEDICAL CONSIDERATIONS
If you have any of the following medical conditions, make sure your doctor is aware of it.

- liver disease or alcoholism—phenelzine levels may be higher than expected
- kidney disease—phenelzine levels may be higher than expected
- heart problems—some heart problems can be worsened by phenelzine. It should not be taken by someone who has had a recent heart attack
- high blood pressure—blood pressure may be increased
- urinary retention, prostate enlargement—urination may become more difficult
- seizure disorder—phenelzine can lower seizure threshold
- diabetes mellitus (sugar diabetes)—blood sugar levels may be affected
- thyroid disorders—phenelzine may cause increased heart rate
- pheochromocytoma—can lead to high blood pressure

Drug Name: PIMOZIDE   (PIM-o-zide)
Drug Category: Neuroleptic; Antipsychotic
Requires prescription

Commonly Used Brand-Name Products
Tablets Orap 2 mg

GENERAL INFORMATION

Effective in treating Tourette's syndrome, to help reduce motor tics and vocalizations. Has been used to treat schizophrenia symptoms.

Before Taking this Medication

Talk to your doctor about the benefits and risks associated with pimozide. Make sure you understand how to take it safely and effectively. Make sure your doctor has the following information in detail:

- any allergic or bad reactions you have had to pimozide or any other medication
- all prescription and over-the-counter medicines you are taking
- your complete medical history
- if you are pregnant, could be pregnant, or are planning a pregnancy in the near future, pimozide has not been shown to be absolutely safe
- if you are breast-feeding, pimozide can pass into breast milk and affect the baby

DOSAGE

<u>Adults and children over 12:</u> 1–10 mg daily. There is a wide effective dosage range. The starting dose will be small and gradually be increased.

<u>Children under 12:</u> Dosages in this age group have not been established.

DIRECTIONS FOR PROPER USE

- *Take exactly as prescribed. Do not take more or less than prescribed.*
- It may take several weeks before you feel the full benefits.

PRECAUTIONS

Alcohol should be avoided while taking pimozide.

Side Effects

Not all side effects will occur. Many side effects will diminish with time. *However, some side effects may be warning signs of toxicity and will require attention from your doctor.* Check with your doctor immediately if you experience any of the following:

- seizure, high fever, fast or irregular heartbeat, very low blood pressure, faintness, any abnormal movements of the mouth, tongue, neck, arms or legs, difficulty speaking or swallowing, imbalance or difficulty walking normally, severe muscle stiffness, discoloration of the skin or eyes, confusion, significant drowsiness, restlessness, difficulty urinating, sexual problems, vomiting, diarrhea, unusual bruising or bleeding, severe skin reaction to sunlight (burning or blistering), severe constipation, breast pain or enlargement

Some side effects appear when you first start taking pimozide and go away for most people. If the following side effects continue, contact your doctor.

- dry mouth, mild to moderate constipation, dizziness, hand tremor, stuffy nose, weight gain

Drug Interactions

Pimozide can adversely interact with the following frequently prescribed medications:

- lithium—increased neurologic side effects
- levodopa—decreased effectiveness of levodopa
- stimulants—pimozide can mask tics caused by stimulants
- anticonvulsants—decreased pimozide levels
- tricyclic antidepressants—increased TCA levels

MEDICAL CONSIDERATIONS

If you have any of the following medical conditions, make sure your doctor is aware of it.

- kidney disease—pimozide levels may be higher than expected
- liver disease—pimozide levels may be higher than expected
- heart problems—some heart problems can be worsened by pimozide
- seizure disorder—pimozide may lower seizure threshold
- urinary retention, prostate enlargement—urination may be more difficult
- glaucoma—pimozide can increase pressure inside the eye
- Parkinson's disease—some Parkinson's symptoms may be worsened
- breast cancer—may increase risk of cancer progression

Drug Name: PROTRIPTYLINE　(pro-TRIP-ti-leen)

Drug Category: Antidepressant, tricyclic
Requires prescription

Commonly Used Brand-Name Products
Tablets Vivactil 5 mg, 10 mg

GENERAL INFORMATION

Highly effective in treating major depression. If used to treat the depressed phase of bipolar disorder, watch for signs of mania or hypomania. Due to the activating effects of protriptyline, it is sometimes used to treat conditions associated with excess sleeping.

Before Taking this Medication

Talk to your doctor about the benefits and risks associated with protriptyline. Make sure you understand how to take it safely and effectively. Make sure your doctor has the following information in detail:

- any allergic or bad reactions you have had to protriptyline or any other medication
- all prescription and over-the-counter medicines you are taking
- your complete medical history
- if you are pregnant, could be pregnant, or are planning a pregnancy in the near future, protriptyline has not been shown to be absolutely safe
- if you are breast-feeding, protriptyline can pass into breast milk and affect the baby

DOSAGE

The starting dose of protriptyline will be low and gradually be increased.

Adults:

Depression: Starting dose 5–10 mg daily. Increased up to 45–60 mg daily over 2 to 3 weeks. Because protriptyline can be activating, some people may need to take it during the day.

Conditions associated with excessive sleeping: 15–20 mg at bedtime.

Adolescents: Adolescents may be more susceptible to heart-related side effects. When used in teenagers, heart function should be monitored.

Children 6–12: Safe use and dosages in this age group have not been established.

Older adults are more susceptible to side effects and generally require lower dosages.

DIRECTIONS FOR PROPER USE

- *Take exactly as prescribed. Do not take more or less than prescribed. Accidental or intended overdoses of protriptyline are potentially fatal.*
- If you miss a dose, do not take it late in the day. It may keep you awake. Do not double doses.
- It may take several weeks before you feel the full benefits.
- Do not abruptly stop taking protriptyline unless instructed to do so by your doctor. Gradually reducing the dose can help prevent mood changes, headache, or diarrhea.

PRECAUTIONS

Alcohol can cause changes in mood and may interfere with protriptyline's effectiveness. *Alcohol should be avoided while taking protriptyline.*

Side Effects

Not all side effects will occur. Many side effects will diminish with time. *However, some side effects may require attention from your doctor.* Check with your doctor immediately if you experience any of the following:

- seizure, changes in blood pressure, irregular heart rate, shortness of breath, problems with urination, (difficult or painful urination; unable to urinate), confusion, extreme sedation, excitation or mania, increased skin sensitivity to sunlight, extreme constipation, yellow skin or eyes

Some side effects appear when you first start taking protriptyline and go away for most people. If the following side effects continue, contact your doctor.

- stimulation, anxiety, insomnia, dizziness, blurred vision, dry mouth, mild to moderate constipation, increased appetite, weight gain, breast enlargement (men or women), discharge from the breast, sexual problems, hand tremor, persistent sore throat

Drug Interactions

Protriptyline can adversely interact with the following frequently prescribed medications:

- cimetidine (Tagamet)—can cause high protriptyline levels
- SSRI antidepressants—can cause high protriptyline levels
- MAOI antidepressants—severe reaction causing dangerously high blood pressure, high body temperature, seizures, or death

- clonidine—if clonidine is being taken for high blood pressure, protriptyline may cause it to work less well
- antipsychotics—may increase certain neurologic side effects
- thyroid hormones—increased effects of both, especially excitation and changes in heart rate or rhythm
- drugs used during surgery—can cause increased blood pressure. Make sure your doctors are aware of upcoming planned surgeries

MEDICAL CONSIDERATIONS
If you have any of the following medical conditions, make sure your doctor is aware of it.

- liver disease or alcoholism—protriptyline levels may be higher than expected
- kidney disease—protriptyline levels may be higher than expected
- glaucoma—protriptyline can increase pressure inside the eye
- heart problems—some heart problems can be worsened by protriptyline. It should not be taken by someone who has had a recent heart attack
- urinary retention, prostate enlargement—urination may become more difficult
- seizure disorder—protriptyline can lower seizure threshold
- diabetes mellitus (sugar diabetes)—blood sugar levels may be affected
- thyroid disorders—protriptyline may cause increased heart rate

---

Drug Name: QUAZEPAM   (KWAY-ze-pam)

Drug Category: Insomnia medicine
Requires prescription, controlled substance, moderate potential for abuse

Commonly Used Brand-Name Products
Tablets Doral 7.5 mg and 15 mg

GENERAL INFORMATION
Highly effective in treating insomnia.

Before Taking this Medication

Talk to your doctor about the benefits and risks associated with quazepam. Make sure you understand how to take it safely and effectively. You and your family members should be very familiar with the side effects and signs of having too much quazepam in your system. Make sure your doctor has the following information in detail:

- any allergic or bad reactions you have had to quazepam or any other medication
- all prescription and over-the-counter medicines you are taking
- your complete medical history
- if you are pregnant, could be pregnant, or are planning a pregnancy in the near future, quazepam should not be taken
- if you are breast-feeding, quazepam can pass into breast milk and affect the baby

DOSAGE

Adults: 7.5 mg to 15 mg at bedtime.

Older adults are more susceptible to side effects and generally require lower dosages.

Children under 18: Safe use has not been established in this age group.

DIRECTIONS FOR PROPER USE

- *Take exactly as prescribed. Do not take more or less than prescribed. Quazepam levels that are too high can cause serious toxicity.*
- If you take quazepam regularly for an extended period of time, do not stop taking it unless told to do so by your doctor. It may be necessary to gradually reduce the dose of quazepam before stopping completely.
- If you miss a dose, take it as soon as possible if it is within one hour of the scheduled time. However, quazepam should be taken only if you are sure you will get a full night's sleep of at least 7 to 8 hours.

PRECAUTIONS

Alcohol should be avoided while taking quazepam.

Side Effects

Not all side effects will occur. Many side effects will diminish with time. *However, some side effects may be warning signs of toxicity and will require attention from your doctor.* Check with your doctor immediately if you experience any of the following:

- confusion, severe drowsiness, slurred speech, severe weakness, unusual thoughts, shortness of breath, excitement, hyperactivity

Some side effects appear when you first start taking quazepam and go away for most people. If the following side effects continue, contact your doctor.

- dizziness, light-headedness, drowsiness, blurred vision

Drug Interactions
Quazepam can adversely interact with the following frequently prescribed medications:

- cimetidine (Tagamet)—can cause high quazepam levels
- disulfiram (Antabuse)—can cause high quazepam levels
- birth control pills—can cause high quazepam levels
- alcohol and other drugs that depress certain functions of the nervous system, when combined with quazepam, can cause extreme drowsiness and slowed reaction times. Examples of these medicines are antihistamines, narcotics, and barbiturates.
- levodopa—decreased effectiveness of levodopa

MEDICAL CONSIDERATIONS
If you have any of the following medical conditions, make sure your doctor is aware of it.

- liver disease or alcoholism—quazepam levels may be higher than expected
- kidney disease—quazepam levels may be higher than expected
- drug dependence or alcohol dependence—dependence on quazepam may occur
- seizure disorder—stopping quazepam abruptly may cause seizures
- chronic lung disease—quazepam may make breathing more difficult

---

Drug Name: QUETIAPINE   (kwe-TIE-a-peen)

Drug Category: Neuroleptic; Antipsychotic
Requires prescription

Commonly Used Brand-Name Products
Tablets Seroquel 25 mg, 100 mg, 200 mg

GENERAL INFORMATION

Highly effective in treating psychotic symptoms, such as hallucinations and delusions. It has been most widely studied in schizophrenia, but may also be useful in treating the psychotic symptoms associated with schizoaffective disorder, bipolar disorder, or major depression with psychotic features.

Before Taking this Medication

Talk to your doctor about the benefits and risks associated with quetiapine. Make sure you understand how to take it safely and effectively. You and your family members should be very familiar with the side effects. Make sure your doctor has the following information in detail:

- any allergic or bad reactions you have had to quetiapine or any other medication
- all prescription and over-the-counter medicines you are taking
- your complete medical history
- if you are pregnant, could be pregnant, or are planning a pregnancy in the near future, quetiapine has not been shown to be absolutely safe
- if you are breast-feeding, quetiapine can pass into breast milk and affect the baby

DOSAGE

Adults:

Psychotic symptoms: 300–750 mg daily.

Older adults are more susceptible to side effects and generally require lower dosages.

Children: Dosages in this age group have not been established.

DIRECTIONS FOR PROPER USE

- *Take exactly as prescribed. Do not take more or less than prescribed.*
- If you miss a dose, take it as soon as possible. However, if the missed dose is within 4 hours of your next dose, skip the missed dose and resume with your next scheduled dose.
- It may take several weeks before you feel the full benefits.

PRECAUTIONS

Alcohol should be avoided while taking quetiapine.

Side Effects

Not all side effects will occur. Many side effects will diminish with time. *However, some side effects may be warning signs of*

toxicity and will require attention from your doctor. Check with your doctor immediately if you experience any of the following:

- seizure, high fever, fast or irregular heartbeat, very low blood pressure, faintness, any abnormal movements of the mouth, tongue, neck, arms or legs, difficulty speaking or swallowing, imbalance or difficulty walking normally, severe muscle stiffness, discoloration of the skin or eyes, confusion, significant drowsiness, restlessness, difficulty urinating, sexual problems, vomiting, diarrhea, unusual bruising or bleeding, severe skin reaction to sunlight (burning or blistering), severe constipation, breast pain or enlargement

Some side effects appear when you first start taking quetiapine and go away for most people. If the following side effects continue, contact your doctor.

- dry mouth, nausea, vomiting, mild to moderate constipation, dizziness, hand tremor, stuffy nose, weight gain

Drug Interactions
Quetiapine can adversely interact with the following frequently prescribed medications:

- lithium—increased neurologic side effects
- levodopa—decreased effectiveness of levodopa
- amphetamines—increased psychotic symptoms are possible
- anticonvulsants—decreased quetiapine levels
- tricyclic antidepressants—increased TCA levels

MEDICAL CONSIDERATIONS
If you have any of the following medical conditions, make sure your doctor is aware of it.

- kidney disease—quetiapine levels may be higher than expected
- liver disease—quetiapine levels may be higher than expected
- heart or blood pressure problems—these can be worsened by quetiapine
- thyroid disease—quetiapine may affect thyroid function

Quetiapine has not been widely studied in people with the following conditions. However, similar medicines are used with caution in the following medical conditions. Make sure your doctor is aware if you have any of the following:

- seizure disorder—possible lower seizure threshold
- urinary retention, prostate enlargement—urination may be more difficult
- glaucoma—may increase pressure inside the eye

- Parkinson's disease—some Parkinson's symptoms may be worsened
- breast cancer—may increase risk of cancer progression

Drug Name: RISPERIDONE   (ris-PAIR-i-doan)

Drug Category: Neuroleptic; Antipsychotic
Requires prescription

Commonly Used Brand-Name Products
Tablets Risperdal 1 mg, 2 mg, 3 mg **Solution** Risperdal 1 mg/ml

GENERAL INFORMATION
Highly effective in treating psychotic symptoms, such as hallucinations and delusions. It has been most widely studied in schizophrenia, but may also be useful in treating the psychotic symptoms associated with schizoaffective disorder, bipolar disorder, or major depression with psychotic features.

Before Taking this Medication
Talk to your doctor about the benefits and risks associated with risperidone. Make sure you understand how to take it safely and effectively. You and your family members should be very familiar with the side effects. Make sure your doctor has the following information in detail:

- any allergic or bad reactions you have had to risperidone or any other medication
- all prescription and over-the-counter medicines you are taking
- your complete medical history
- if you are pregnant, could be pregnant, or are planning a pregnancy in the near future, risperidone has not been shown to be absolutely safe
- if you are breast-feeding, risperidone can pass into breast milk and affect the baby

DOSAGE
Adults:
  Psychotic symptoms: 2–16 mg daily.

<u>Older adults</u> are more susceptible to side effects and generally require lower dosages.

<u>Children:</u> Dosages in this age group have not been established.

DIRECTIONS FOR PROPER USE

- *Take exactly as prescribed. Do not take more or less than prescribed.*
- If you miss a dose, take it as soon as possible. However, if the missed dose is within 4 hours of your next dose, skip the missed dose and resume with your next scheduled dose.
- It may take several weeks before you feel the full benefits.

PRECAUTIONS

Alcohol should be avoided while taking risperidone.

Side Effects

Not all side effects will occur. Many side effects will diminish with time. *However, some side effects may be warning signs of toxicity and will require attention from your doctor.* Check with your doctor immediately if you experience any of the following:

- seizure, high fever, fast or irregular heartbeat, very low blood pressure, faintness, any abnormal movements of the mouth, tongue, neck, arms or legs, difficulty speaking or swallowing, imbalance or difficulty walking normally, severe muscle stiffness, discoloration of the skin or eyes, confusion, significant drowsiness, restlessness, difficulty urinating, sexual problems, vomiting, diarrhea, unusual bruising or bleeding, severe skin reaction to sunlight (burning or blistering), severe constipation, breast pain or enlargement

Some side effects appear when you first start taking risperidone and go away for most people. If the following side effects continue, contact your doctor.

- dry mouth, nausea, vomiting, mild to moderate constipation, dizziness, hand tremor, stuffy nose, weight gain

Drug Interactions

Risperidone can adversely interact with the following frequently prescribed medications:

- lithium—increased neurologic side effects
- levodopa—decreased effectiveness of levodopa
- amphetamines—increased psychotic symptoms are possible
- anticonvulsants—decreased risperidone levels
- tricyclic antidepressants—increased TCA levels

MEDICAL CONSIDERATIONS

If you have any of the following medical conditions, make sure your doctor is aware of it.

- kidney disease—risperidone levels may be higher than expected
- liver disease—risperidone levels may be higher than expected
- heart problems—some heart problems may be worsened by risperidone
- seizure disorder—risperidone can lower seizure threshold
- urinary retention, prostate enlargement—urination may be more difficult
- glaucoma—risperidone can increase pressure inside the eye
- Parkinson's disease—some Parkinson's symptoms may be worsened
- breast cancer—may increase risk of cancer progression

Drug Name: SERTRALINE   (sur-TRA-leen)

Drug Category: Antidepressant, SSRI
(serotonin specific reuptake inhibitor)
Requires prescription

Commonly Used Brand-Name Products
Tablets Zoloft 50 mg, 100 mg

GENERAL INFORMATION

Highly effective in treating major depression and the depressed phase of bipolar disorder. May be effective in treating obsessive compulsive disorder (OCD), and panic disorder. May be used to treat attention deficit hyperactivity disorder, especially in adults. May be useful in treating bulimia.

Before Taking this Medication

Talk to your doctor about the benefits and risks associated with sertraline. Make sure you understand how to take it safely and effectively. Make sure your doctor has the following information in detail:

- any allergic or bad reactions you have had to sertraline or any other medication
- all prescription and over-the-counter medicines you are taking

- your complete medical history
- if you are pregnant, could be pregnant, or are planning a pregnancy in the near future, sertraline has not been shown to be absolutely safe
- if you are breast-feeding, sertraline can pass into breast milk and affect the baby

DOSAGE
Adults:
    Depression, panic disorder, bulimia: 50–200 mg daily. Dosage increases should not be made more often than every 1 to 2 weeks.
    OCD: 100–200 mg daily.
Children and Adolescents: Safe use has not been established.
Older adults are more susceptible to side effects and generally require lower dosages.

DIRECTIONS FOR PROPER USE
- *Take exactly as prescribed. Do not take more or less than prescribed.*
- Sertraline may be taken on an empty stomach, or with food or meals to lessen stomach upset. It is important, however, to take it the same way every day.
- If you miss a dose, do not try to make it up. Wait and take your next scheduled dose. Do not double doses.
- It may take several weeks before you feel the full benefits.
- Do not abruptly stop taking sertraline unless instructed to do so by your doctor.

PRECAUTIONS
Alcohol can cause changes in mood and may interfere with sertraline's effectiveness. *Alcohol should be avoided while taking sertraline.*

Side Effects
Not all side effects will occur. Many side effects will diminish with time. *However, some side effects may require attention from your doctor.* Check with your doctor immediately if you experience any of the following:
- skin rash or hives, shortness of breath, chills or fever, swelling of the hands or feet, seizures, sore throat

Some side effects appear when you first start taking sertraline and go away for most people. If the following side effects continue, contact your doctor.

- stimulation, anxiety, insomnia, dizziness, sexual problems, sweating, blurred vision, dry mouth, mild to moderate constipation, change in appetite, change in weight, hand tremor, headache

Drug Interactions
Sertraline can adversely interact with the following frequently prescribed medications:

- anticoagulants (blood thinners)—the effect of the anticoagulant can be increased
- some nonsedating antihistamines—cardiac (heart) toxicity
- diet pills—severe reaction causing dangerously high blood pressure, high body temperature, seizures, or death
- cimetidine (Tagamet)—can cause high sertraline levels
- TCA antidepressants—can cause high TCA levels
- MAOI antidepressants—severe reaction causing dangerously high blood pressure, high body temperature, seizures, or death
- antipsychotics—may increase certain neurologic side effects
- lithium—increased lithium levels may cause confusion, dizziness, tremor
- anticonvulsants—increased anticonvulsant levels or decreased sertraline levels

MEDICAL CONSIDERATIONS
If you have any of the following medical conditions, make sure your doctor is aware of it.

- liver disease or alcoholism—sertraline levels may be higher than expected
- kidney disease—sertraline levels may be higher than expected
- seizure disorder—sertraline can lower seizure threshold
- diabetes mellitus (sugar diabetes)—blood sugar levels may be affected

---

Drug Name: TEMAZEPAM   (tem-AZ-e-pam)

Drug Category: Insomnia medicine
Requires prescription, controlled substance, moderate potential for abuse

Commonly Used Brand-Name Products
Capsules Restoril (and generic) 7.5 mg, 15 mg and 30 mg

GENERAL INFORMATION
Highly effective in treating insomnia.

Before Taking this Medication
Talk to your doctor about the benefits and risks associated with temazepam. Make sure you understand how to take it safely and effectively. You and your family members should be very familiar with the side effects and signs of having too much temazepam in your system. Make sure your doctor has the following information in detail:

- any allergic or bad reactions you have had to temazepam or any other medication
- all prescription and over-the-counter medicines you are taking
- your complete medical history
- if you are pregnant, could be pregnant, or are planning a pregnancy in the near future, temazepam should not be taken.
- if you are breast-feeding, temazepam can pass into breast milk and affect the baby

DOSAGE
Adults: 15 mg to 30 mg at bedtime.
Older adults are more susceptible to side effects and generally require lower dosages.
Children under 18: Safe use has not been established in this age group.

DIRECTIONS FOR PROPER USE
- *Take exactly as prescribed. Do not take more or less than prescribed. Temazepam levels that are too high can cause serious toxicity.*
- If you take temazepam regularly for an extended period of time, do not stop taking it unless told to do so by your doctor. It may be necessary to gradually reduce the dose before stopping completely.
- If you miss a dose, take it as soon as possible if it is within one hour of the scheduled time. However, temazepam should be taken only if you are sure you will get a full night's sleep of at least 7 to 8 hours.

PRECAUTIONS
Alcohol should be avoided while taking temazepam.

Side Effects
Not all side effects will occur. Many side effects will diminish with time. *However, some side effects may be warning signs of toxicity and will require attention from your doctor.* Check with your doctor immediately if you experience any of the following:

- confusion, severe drowsiness, slurred speech, severe weakness, unusual thoughts, shortness of breath, excitement, hyperactivity

Some side effects appear when you first start taking temazepam and go away for most people. If the following side effects continue, contact your doctor.

- dizziness, light-headedness, drowsiness, blurred vision

Drug Interactions
Temazepam can adversely interact with the following frequently prescribed medications:

- cimetidine (Tagamet)—can cause high temazepam levels
- disulfiram (Antabuse)—can cause high temazepam levels
- birth control pills—can cause high temazepam levels
- alcohol and other drugs that depress certain functions of the nervous system, when combined with temazepam, cause extreme drowsiness and slowed reaction times. Examples of these medicines are antihistamines, narcotics, and barbiturates.
- levodopa—decreased effectiveness of levodopa

MEDICAL CONSIDERATIONS
If you have any of the following medical conditions, make sure your doctor is aware of it.

- liver disease or alcoholism—temazepam levels may be higher than expected
- kidney disease—temazepam levels may be higher than expected
- drug dependence or alcohol dependence—dependence on temazepam may occur
- seizure disorder—stopping temazepam abruptly may cause seizures
- chronic lung disease—temazepam may make breathing more difficult

Drug Name: THIORIDAZINE   (thi-o-RID-a-zeen))

Drug Category: Neuroleptic; Antipsychotic
Requires prescription

Commonly Used Brand-Name Products
Tablets Mellaril (and generic) 10 mg, 15 mg, 25 mg, 50 mg, 100 mg, 150 mg, 200 mg **Liquids** Solution: Mellaril (and generic) 30 mg/ml and 100 mg/ml Suspension: Mellaril S 25 mg/teaspoonful and 100 mg/teaspoonful

GENERAL INFORMATION
Highly effective in treating psychotic symptoms, such as hallucinations and delusions. These symptoms occur in schizophrenia, schizoaffective disorder, bipolar disorder, or major depression with psychotic features. Also can be used for the short-term management of aggressive, out-of-control behaviors or feelings of anger and rage, and to help with symptoms of anxiety and insomnia.

Before Taking this Medication
Talk to your doctor about the benefits and risks associated with thioridazine. Make sure you understand how to take it safely and effectively. You and your family members should be very familiar with the side effects. Make sure your doctor has the following information in detail:

- any allergic or bad reactions you have had to thioridazine or any other medication
- all prescription and over-the-counter medicines you are taking
- your complete medical history
- if you are pregnant, could be pregnant, or are planning a pregnancy in the near future, thioridazine has not been shown to be absolutely safe
- if you are breast-feeding, thioridazine can pass into breast milk and affect the baby

DOSAGE
Adults and adolescents over 12:
   Psychotic symptoms: 50–800 mg daily. There is a wide effective dosage range.

Anxiety and insomnia: 10–25 mg daily, usually at bedtime, but in extreme anxiety can be given during waking hours.

Older adults are more susceptible to side effects and generally require lower dosages.

Children 2-12: Dosages are based on weight.

Children under 2: Safe use in this age group has not been established.

DIRECTIONS FOR PROPER USE

- *Take exactly as prescribed. Do not take more or less than prescribed.*
- If you take the solution form, the dose must be mixed in water or orange or grapefruit juice before being taken.
- If you miss a dose, take it as soon as possible. However, if the missed dose is within 4 hours of your next dose, skip the missed dose and resume with your next scheduled dose.
- If you are taking the liquid form, avoid contact of the skin with medicine. Irritation can result by the medicine coming into contact with skin. Do not use the liquid form if it becomes discolored or has a sediment at the bottom of the bottle.
- It may take several weeks before you feel the full benefits.

PRECAUTIONS

Alcohol should be avoided while taking thioridazine.

Side Effects

Not all side effects will occur. Many side effects will diminish with time. *However, some side effects may be warning signs of toxicity and will require attention from your doctor.* Check with your doctor immediately if you experience any of the following:

- seizure, high fever, fast or irregular heartbeat, very low blood pressure, faintness, any abnormal movements of the mouth, tongue, neck, arms or legs, difficulty speaking or swallowing, imbalance or difficulty walking normally, severe muscle stiffness, discoloration of the skin or eyes, confusion, significant drowsiness, restlessness, difficulty urinating, sexual problems, vomiting, diarrhea, unusual bruising or bleeding, severe skin reaction to sunlight (burning or blistering), severe constipation, breast pain or enlargement

Some side effects appear when you first start taking thioridazine and go away for most people. If the following side effects continue, contact your doctor.

- dry mouth, mild to moderate constipation, dizziness, hand tremor, stuffy nose, weight gain

Drug Interactions
Thioridazine can adversely interact with the following frequently prescribed medications:

- lithium—increased neurologic side effects
- levodopa—decreased effectiveness of levodopa
- amphetamines—increased psychotic symptoms are possible
- anticonvulsants—decreased thioridazine levels
- tricyclic antidepressants—increased TCA levels

MEDICAL CONSIDERATIONS
If you have any of the following medical conditions, make sure your doctor is aware of it.

- kidney disease—thioridazine levels may be higher than expected
- liver disease—thioridazine levels may be higher than expected
- heart problems—some heart problems can be worsened by thioridazine
- seizure disorder—thioridazine can lower seizure threshold
- urinary retention, prostate enlargement—urination may be more difficult
- glaucoma—thioridazine can increase pressure inside the eye
- Parkinson's disease—some Parkinson's symptoms may be worsened
- breast cancer—may increase risk of cancer progression

Drug Name: THIOTHIXENE   (thi-o-THIX-een)

Drug Category: Neuroleptic; Antipsychotic
Requires prescription

Commonly Used Brand-Name Products	
Capsules Navane (and generic) 1 mg, 2 mg, 5 mg, 10 mg **Liquid** Navane solution 5 mg/ml (contains alcohol)	**Injection** Navane, 2 mg/ml and 5 mg/ml

GENERAL INFORMATION
Highly effective in treating psychotic symptoms, such as hallucinations and delusions. These symptoms occur in schizophrenia, schizoaffective disorder, bipolar disorder, or major depression with psychotic features. Also can be used for the short-term management of aggressive, out-of-control behaviors or feelings of anger and rage, and to help with symptoms of anxiety and insomnia.

Before Taking this Medication
Talk to your doctor about the benefits and risks associated with thiothixene. Make sure you understand how to take it safely and effectively. You and your family members should be very familiar with the side effects. Make sure your doctor has the following information in detail:

- any allergic or bad reactions you have had to thiothixene or any other medication
- all prescription and over-the-counter medicines you are taking
- your complete medical history
- if you are pregnant, could be pregnant, or are planning a pregnancy in the near future, thiothixene has not been shown to be absolutely safe
- if you are breast-feeding, thiothixene can pass into breast milk and affect the baby

DOSAGE
<u>Adults and adolescents:</u>
   <u>Psychotic symptoms:</u> 5–60 mg daily. There is a wide effective dosage range.
   <u>Anxiety and insomnia:</u> 2–5 mg daily, usually at bedtime, but in extreme anxiety can be given during waking hours.
<u>Older adults</u> are more susceptible to side effects and generally require lower dosages.

Children under 12: Dosages in this age group have not been established.

DIRECTIONS FOR PROPER USE

- *Take exactly as prescribed. Do not take more or less than prescribed.*
- If you take the liquid form it must be diluted before swallowing. It may diluted in water, milk, tomato or fruit juice. The dose should be measured carefully.
- If you take the solution form, avoid contact of the skin with the medicine. Irritation can result by the medicine coming into contact with skin. Do not use the liquid form if it becomes very discolored (dark yellow) or has a sediment at the bottom of the bottle.
- If you miss a dose, take it as soon as possible. However, if the missed dose is within 4 hours of your next dose, skip the missed dose and resume with your next scheduled dose.
- It may take several weeks before you feel the full benefits.

PRECAUTIONS

Alcohol should be avoided while taking thiothixene.

Side Effects

Not all side effects will occur. Many side effects will diminish with time. *However, some side effects may be warning signs of toxicity and will require attention from your doctor.* Check with your doctor immediately if you experience any of the following:

- seizure, high fever, fast or irregular heartbeat, very low blood pressure, faintness, any abnormal movements of the mouth, tongue, neck, arms or legs, difficulty speaking or swallowing, imbalance or difficulty walking normally, severe muscle stiffness, discoloration of the skin or eyes, confusion, significant drowsiness, restlessness, difficulty urinating, sexual problems, vomiting, diarrhea, unusual bruising or bleeding, severe skin reaction to sunlight (burning or blistering), severe constipation, breast pain or enlargement

Some side effects appear when you first start taking thiothixene and go away for most people. If the following side effects continue, contact your doctor.

- dry mouth, mild to moderate constipation, dizziness, hand tremor, stuffy nose, weight gain

Drug Interactions

Thiothixene can adversely interact with the following frequently prescribed medications:

- lithium—increased neurologic side effects
- levodopa—decreased effectiveness of levodopa
- amphetamines—increased psychotic symptoms are possible
- anticonvulsants—decreased thiothixene levels
- tricyclic antidepressants—increased TCA levels

MEDICAL CONSIDERATIONS

If you have any of the following medical conditions, make sure your doctor is aware of it.

- kidney disease—thiothixene levels may be higher than expected
- liver disease—thiothixene levels may be higher than expected
- heart problems—some heart problems can be worsened by thiothixene
- seizure disorder—thiothixene can lower seizure threshold
- urinary retention, prostate enlargement—urination may be more difficult
- glaucoma—thiothixene can increase pressure inside the eye
- Parkinson's disease—some Parkinson's symptoms may be worsened
- breast cancer—may increase risk of cancer progression

Drug Name: TRANYLCYPROMINE   (tran-el-SIGH-pro-meen)

Drug Category: Antidepressant, MAOI (monoamine oxidase inhibitor)
Requires prescription

Commonly Used Brand-Name Products
Tablets Parnate 10 mg

GENERAL INFORMATION

Highly effective in treating major depression, and the depressed phase of bipolar disorder. Very effective in treating panic disorder. Effective in treating social phobia.

Before Taking this Medication

Talk to your doctor about the benefits and risks associated with tranylcypromine. Make sure you understand how to take it safely and effectively. Make sure your doctor has the following information in detail:

- any allergic or bad reactions you have had to tranylcypromine or any other medication
- all prescription and over-the-counter medicines you are taking
- your complete medical history
- if you are pregnant, could be pregnant, or are planning a pregnancy in the near future, tranylcypromine has not been shown to be absolutely safe.
- if you are breast-feeding, tranylcypromine can pass into breast milk and affect the baby

DOSAGE

The starting dose of tranylcypromine will be low and gradually be increased.

<u>Adults:</u> 20–40 mg daily.

<u>Older adults</u> are more susceptible to side effects and generally require lower dosages.

<u>Children under 16:</u> Safe use and dosages in this age group have not been established.

DIRECTIONS FOR PROPER USE

- *Take exactly as prescribed. Do not take more or less than prescribed. Accidental or intended overdoses of tranylcypromine are potentially fatal.*
- *Follow the dietary instructions described below carefully while taking tranylcypromine. Not doing so can lead to dangerously high blood pressure.*
- The amount of tyramine, or tryptophan, in your diet must be restricted while taking tranylcypromine. Tyramine is found in foods that have been aged, preserved, or that have undergone protein breakdown. The amount of tyramine in food is **not** inactivated by cooking. These restrictions will need to be followed for two weeks after tranylcypromine has been stopped. (See "Foods to Avoid Completely" in chapter 5 on page 63.)
- *Check with your doctor or pharmacist before taking any other prescription or over-the-counter medicine.*
- It is advised that you check your blood pressure frequently while taking tranylcypromine.

- If you miss a bedtime dose, do not take it the next morning. It may make you drowsy. Do not double doses.
- It may take several weeks before you feel the full benefits.
- Do not abruptly stop taking tranylcypromine unless instructed to do so by your doctor. Gradually reducing the dose can help prevent mood changes, headache, or diarrhea.

PRECAUTIONS
Alcohol can cause changes in mood and may interfere with tranylcypromine's effectiveness. *Alcohol should be avoided while taking tranylcypromine.*

Side Effects
Not all side effects will occur. Many side effects will diminish with time. *However, some side effects may require attention from your doctor.* Check with your doctor immediately if you experience any of the following:

- seizure, changes in blood pressure, severe headache, irregular heart rate, shortness of breath, problems with urination, (difficult or painful urination; unable to urinate), confusion, extreme sedation, excitation or mania, extreme sweating, severe skin sensitivity to sunlight (burning or blistering), extreme constipation, yellow skin or eyes

Some side effects appear when you first start taking tranylcypromine and go away for most people. If the following side effects continue, contact your doctor.

- dizziness, blurred vision, dry mouth, mild to moderate constipation, increased appetite, weight gain, hand tremor

Drug Interactions
Tranylcypromine can adversely interact with the following frequently prescribed medications. A severe reaction causing dangerously high blood pressure, high body temperature, seizures, or death is possible. These interactions are possible for up to 2 weeks after tranylcypromine has been stopped. A "washout" period of up to 5 weeks after stopping some of the medications listed below may be necessary before starting tranylcypromine.

- SSRI antidepressants
- TCA antidepressants
- stimulant drugs—amphetamines, methylphenidate (Ritalin), cocaine
- ephedrine, pseudoephedrine—found in prescription and over-the-counter cough, cold, or asthma medicines

- phenylephrine, phenylpropanolamine—found in prescription and over-the-counter cough, cold, or asthma medicines
- levodopa
- buspirone (Buspar)
- dextromethorphan—found in prescription and over-the-counter cough syrups and lozenges
- meperidine (Demerol)

MEDICAL CONSIDERATIONS

If you have any of the following medical conditions, make sure your doctor is aware of it.

- liver disease or alcoholism—tranylcypromine levels may be higher than expected
- kidney disease—tranylcypromine levels may be higher than expected
- heart problems—some heart problems can be worsened by tranylcypromine. It should not be taken by someone who has had a recent heart attack
- high blood pressure—blood pressure may be increased
- urinary retention, prostate enlargement—urination may become more difficult
- seizure disorder—tranylcypromine can lower seizure threshold
- diabetes mellitus (sugar diabetes)—blood sugar levels may be affected
- thyroid disorders—tranylcypromine may cause increased heart rate
- pheochromocytoma—can lead to high blood pressure

Drug Name: TRAZODONE   (TRAZ-oh-doan)

Drug Category: Antidepressant, atypical
Requires prescription

Commonly Used Brand-Name Products
Tablets
Desyrel (and generic) 50 mg, 100 mg, 150 mg, 300 mg

GENERAL INFORMATION

Highly effective in treating major depression and the depressed phase of bipolar disorder. Due to its sedative effects, it is sometimes given in low doses to help with anxiety and insomnia. It is also used to treat certain chronic pain disorders, such as migraine headache and diabetic neuropathy.

Before Taking this Medication

Talk to your doctor about the benefits and risks associated with trazodone. Make sure you understand how to take it safely and effectively. Make sure your doctor has the following information in detail:

- any allergic or bad reactions you have had to trazodone or any other medication
- all prescription and over-the-counter medicines you are taking
- your complete medical history
- if you are pregnant, could be pregnant, or are planning a pregnancy in the near future, trazodone has not been shown to be absolutely safe
- if you are breast-feeding, trazodone can pass into breast milk and affect the baby

DOSAGE

The starting dose of trazodone will be low and gradually be increased.

Adults:

Depression: Starting dose 50 mg at bedtime. Increased to 75–500 mg at bedtime over 2 to 3 weeks.

Insomnia: 50–100 mg at bedtime.

Chronic pain syndromes: 50–100 mg daily.

Older adults are more susceptible to side effects and generally require lower dosages.

Children and adolescents under 18: Safe use and dosages in this age group have not been established.

DIRECTIONS FOR PROPER USE

- *Take exactly as prescribed. Do not take more or less than prescribed. Accidental or intended overdoses of trazodone are potentially fatal.*
- Take with food or milk to lessen stomach upset.
- If you miss a bedtime dose, do not take it the next morning. It may make you drowsy. Do not double doses.
- It may take several weeks before you feel the full benefits.
- Do not abruptly stop taking trazodone unless instructed to do so by your doctor. Gradually reducing the dose can help prevent mood changes, headache, or diarrhea.

PRECAUTIONS

Alcohol can cause changes in mood and may interfere with trazodone's effectiveness. *Alcohol should be avoided while taking trazodone.*

Side Effects

Not all side effects will occur. Many side effects will diminish with time. *However, some side effects may require attention from your doctor.* Check with your doctor immediately if you experience any of the following:

- seizure, prolonged erection of the penis (considered a medical emergency), changes in blood pressure, irregular heart rate, shortness of breath, problems with urination, (difficult or painful urination; unable to urinate), confusion, extreme sedation, excitation or mania, increased skin sensitivity to sunlight, extreme constipation, yellow skin or eyes

Some side effects appear when you first start taking trazodone and go away for most people. If the following side effects continue, contact your doctor.

- dizziness, blurred vision, dry mouth, mild to moderate constipation, increased appetite, weight gain, breast enlargement (men or women), discharge from the breast, sexual problems, hand tremor, persistent sore throat

Drug Interactions

Trazodone can adversely interact with the following frequently prescribed medications:

- SSRI antidepressants—can cause high trazodone levels
- MAOI antidepressants—severe reaction causing dangerously high blood pressure, high body temperature, seizures, or death
- clonidine—if clonidine is being taken for high blood pressure, trazodone may cause it to work less well
- antipsychotics—may increase certain neurologic side effects
- drugs used during surgery—can cause increased blood pressure. Make sure your doctors are aware of upcoming planned surgeries

MEDICAL CONSIDERATIONS

If you have any of the following medical conditions, make sure your doctor is aware of it.

- liver disease or alcoholism—trazodone levels may be higher than expected
- kidney disease—trazodone levels may be higher than expected

- heart problems—some heart problems can be worsened by trazodone. It should not be taken by someone who has had a recent heart attack
- urinary retention, prostate enlargement—urination may become more difficult

---

Drug Name: TRIAZOLAM (try-AZ-o-lam)

Drug Category: Insomnia medicine

Requires prescription, controlled substance, moderate to high potential for abuse

Commonly Used Brand-Name Products
Tablets
Halcion 0.125 mg and 0.25 mg

GENERAL INFORMATION

Highly effective in treating insomnia.

Before Taking this Medication

Talk to your doctor about the benefits and risks associated with triazolam. Make sure you understand how to take it safely and effectively. You and your family members should be very familiar with the side effects and signs of having too much triazolam in your system. Make sure your doctor has the following information in detail:

- any allergic or bad reactions you have had to triazolam or any other medication
- all prescription and over-the-counter medicines you are taking
- your complete medical history
- if you are pregnant, could be pregnant, or are planning a pregnancy in the near future, triazolam should not be taken
- if you are breast-feeding, triazolam can pass into breast milk and affect the baby

DOSAGE

Adults: 0.125 mg to 0.25 mg at bedtime.

Older adults are more susceptible to side effects and generally require lower dosages.

Children under 18: Safe use has not been established in this age group.

DIRECTIONS FOR PROPER USE

- *Take exactly as prescribed. Do not take more or less than prescribed. Triazolam levels that are too high can cause serious toxicity. Triazolam may cause more serious side effects than other medications of this type. Close monitoring by a physician is necessary for safe use of this medicine.*
- If you take triazolam regularly for an extended period of time, do not stop taking it unless told to do so by your doctor. It may be necessary to gradually reduce the dose before stopping completely.
- If you miss a dose, take it as soon as possible if it is within one hour of the scheduled time. However, triazolam should be taken only if you are sure you will get a full night's sleep of at least 7 to 8 hours.

PRECAUTIONS

Alcohol should be avoided while taking triazolam.

Side Effects

Not all side effects will occur. Many side effects will diminish with time. *However, some side effects may be warning signs of toxicity and will require attention from your doctor.* Check with your doctor immediately if you experience any of the following:

- confusion, severe drowsiness, slurred speech, severe weakness, unusual thoughts, shortness of breath, excitement, hyperactivity, unusual behaviors, significant memory problems

Some side effects appear when you first start taking triazolam and go away for most people. If the following side effects continue, contact your doctor.

- dizziness, light-headedness, drowsiness, blurred vision

Drug Interactions

Triazolam can adversely interact with the following frequently prescribed medications:

- cimetidine (Tagamet)—can cause high triazolam levels
- disulfiram (Antabuse)—can cause high triazolam levels
- birth control pills—can cause high triazolam levels
- alcohol and other drugs that depress certain functions of the nervous system, when combined with triazolam, can cause extreme drowsiness and slowed reaction times. Examples of these medicines are antihistamines, narcotics, and barbiturates
- levodopa—decreased effectiveness of levodopa

MEDICAL CONSIDERATIONS

If you have any of the following medical conditions, make sure your doctor is aware of it.

- liver disease or alcoholism—triazolam levels may be higher than expected
- kidney disease—triazolam levels may be higher than expected
- drug dependence or alcohol dependence—dependence on triazolam may occur
- seizure disorder—stopping triazolam abruptly may cause seizures
- chronic lung disease—triazolam may make breathing more difficult

---

Drug Name: TRIFLUOPERAZINE   (tri-FLEW-o-pair-a-zeen)

Drug Category: Neuroleptic; Antipsychotic
Requires prescription

Commonly Used Brand-Name Products	
Tablets Stelazine (and generic) 1 mg, 2 mg, 5 mg, 10 mg **Liquid** Stelazine (and generic) 10 mg/ml	**Injection** Stelazine (and generic) 2 mg/ml

GENERAL INFORMATION

Highly effective in treating psychotic symptoms, such as hallucinations and delusions. These symptoms occur in schizophrenia, schizoaffective disorder, bipolar disorder, or major depression with psychotic features. Also can be used for the short-term management of aggressive, out-of-control behaviors or feelings of anger and rage, and to help with symptoms of anxiety and insomnia.

Before Taking this Medication

Talk to your doctor about the benefits and risks associated with trifluoperazine. Make sure you understand how to take it safely and effectively. You and your family members should be very familiar with the side effects. Make sure your doctor has the following information in detail:

- any allergic or bad reactions you have had to trifluoperazine or any other medication
- all prescription and over-the-counter medicines you are taking
- your complete medical history
- if you are pregnant, could be pregnant, or are planning a pregnancy in the near future, trifluoperazine has not been shown to be absolutely safe
- if you are breast-feeding, trifluoperazine can pass into breast milk and affect the baby

DOSAGE
Adults and adolescents:
  Psychotic symptoms: 5–80 mg daily. There is a wide effective dosage range.
  Anxiety and insomnia: 2–5 mg daily, usually at bedtime, but in extreme anxiety can be given during waking hours.
Older adults are more susceptible to side effects and generally require lower dosages.
Children 6-12: Dosage is based on weight.
Children under 6: Dosages in this age group have not been established.

DIRECTIONS FOR PROPER USE
- *Take exactly as prescribed. Do not take more or less than prescribed.*
- If you take the liquid form, the dose must be mixed in water, milk, tomato or fruit juice before swallowing. Measure the dose carefully.
- If you take the solution form, avoid contact of the skin with the medicine. Irritation can result by the medicine coming into contact with skin. Do not use the liquid form if it becomes very discolored (dark yellow) or has a sediment at the bottom of the bottle.
- If you miss a dose, take it as soon as possible. However, if the missed dose is within 4 hours of your next dose, skip the missed dose and resume with your next scheduled dose.
- It may take several weeks before you feel the full benefits.

PRECAUTIONS
Alcohol should be avoided while taking trifluoperazine.

Side Effects
Not all side effects will occur. Many side effects will diminish with time. *However, some side effects may be warning signs of*

toxicity and will require attention from your doctor. Check with your doctor immediately if you experience any of the following:

- seizure, high fever, fast or irregular heartbeat, very low blood pressure, faintness, any abnormal movements of the mouth, tongue, neck, arms or legs, difficulty speaking or swallowing, imbalance or difficulty walking normally, severe muscle stiffness, discoloration of the skin or eyes, confusion, significant drowsiness, restlessness, difficulty urinating, sexual problems, vomiting, diarrhea, unusual bruising or bleeding, severe skin reaction to sunlight (burning or blistering), severe constipation, breast pain or enlargement

Some side effects appear when you first start taking trifluoperazine and go away for most people. If the following side effects continue, contact your doctor.

- dry mouth, mild to moderate constipation, dizziness, hand tremor, stuffy nose, weight gain

Drug Interactions

Trifluoperazine can adversely interact with the following frequently prescribed medications:

- lithium—increased neurologic side effects
- levodopa—decreased effectiveness of levodopa
- amphetamines—increased psychotic symptoms are possible
- anticonvulsants—decreased trifluoperazine levels
- tricyclic antidepressants—increased TCA levels

MEDICAL CONSIDERATIONS

If you have any of the following medical conditions, make sure your doctor is aware of it.

- kidney disease—trifluoperazine levels may be higher than expected
- liver disease—trifluoperazine levels may be higher than expected
- heart problems—some heart problems can be worsened by trifluoperazine
- seizure disorder—trifluoperazine can lower seizure threshold
- urinary retention, prostate enlargement—urination may be more difficult
- glaucoma—trifluoperazine can increase pressure inside the eye
- Parkinson's disease—some Parkinson's symptoms may be worsened
- breast cancer—may increase risk of cancer progression

Drug Name: TRIMIPRAMINE   (try-MIP-ra-meen)

Drug Category: Antidepressant, tricyclic
Requires prescription

Commonly Used Brand-Name Products
Capsules Surmontil (and generic) 25 mg, 50 mg, 100 mg

GENERAL INFORMATION
Highly effective in treating major depression and the depressed phase of bipolar disorder. Also used to treat certain chronic pain disorders, such as migraine headache and diabetic neuropathy.

Before Taking this Medication
Talk to your doctor about the benefits and risks associated with trimipramine. Make sure you understand how to take it safely and effectively. Make sure your doctor has the following information in detail:

- any allergic or bad reactions you have had to trimipramine or any other medication
- all prescription and over-the-counter medicines you are taking
- your complete medical history
- if you are pregnant, could be pregnant, or are planning a pregnancy in the near future, trimipramine has not been shown to be absolutely safe
- if you are breast-feeding, trimipramine can pass into breast milk and affect the baby

DOSAGE
The starting dose of trimipramine will be low and gradually be increased.
Adults:
  Depression: Starting dose 25–50 mg at bedtime. Increased to 75—300 mg at bedtime over 2 to 3 weeks.
  Chronic pain syndromes: 50–100 mg daily.
Adolescents: Adolescents may be more susceptible to heart-related side effects. Heart function should be monitored.
Children up to 12: Safe use and dosages in this age group have not been established.
Older adults are more susceptible to side effects and generally require lower dosages.

DIRECTIONS FOR PROPER USE

- *Take exactly as prescribed. Do not take more or less than pre-scribed. Accidental or intended overdoses of trimipramine are potentially fatal.*
- If you miss a bedtime dose, do not take it the next morning. It may make you drowsy. Do not double doses.
- It may take several weeks before you feel the full benefits.
- Do not abruptly stop taking trimipramine unless instructed to do so by your doctor. Gradually reducing the dose can help prevent mood changes, headache, or diarrhea.

PRECAUTIONS

Alcohol can cause changes in mood and may interfere with trimipramine's effectiveness. *Alcohol should be avoided while taking trimipramine.*

Side Effects

Not all side effects will occur. Many side effects will diminish with time. *However, some side effects may require attention from your doctor.* Check with your doctor immediately if you experience any of the following:

- seizure, changes in blood pressure, irregular heart rate, shortness of breath, problems with urination, (difficult or painful urination; unable to urinate), confusion, extreme sedation, excitation or mania, severe skin sensitivity to sunlight (burning or blistering), extreme constipation, yellow skin or eyes

Some side effects appear when you first start taking trimipramine and go away for most people. If the following side effects continue, contact your doctor.

- dizziness, blurred vision, dry mouth, mild to moderate constipation, increased appetite, weight gain, breast enlargement (men or women), discharge from the breast, sexual problems, hand tremor, persistent sore throat

Drug Interactions

Trimipramine can adversely interact with the following frequently prescribed medications:

- cimetidine (Tagamet)—can cause high trimipramine levels
- SSRI antidepressants—can cause high trimipramine levels
- MAOI antidepressants—severe reaction causing dangerously high blood pressure, high body temperature, seizures, or death
- clonidine—if clonidine is being taken for high blood pressure, trimipramine may cause it to work less well

- antipsychotics—may increase certain neurologic side effects
- thyroid hormones—increased effects of both, especially excitation and changes in heart rate or rhythm
- drugs used during surgery—can cause increased blood pressure. Make sure your doctors are aware of upcoming planned surgeries

MEDICAL CONSIDERATIONS

If you have any of the following medical conditions, make sure your doctor is aware of it.

- liver disease or alcoholism—trimipramine levels may be higher than expected
- kidney disease—trimipramine levels may be higher than expected
- glaucoma—trimipramine can increase pressure inside the eye
- heart problems—some heart problems can be worsened by trimipramine. It should not be taken by someone who has had a recent heart attack
- urinary retention, prostate enlargement—urination may become more difficult
- seizure disorder—trimipramine can lower seizure threshold
- diabetes mellitus (sugar diabetes)—blood sugar levels may be affected
- thyroid disorders—trimipramine may cause increased heart rate

---

Drug Name: VALPROATE   (val-PRO-ate)

Drug Category: Mood stabilizer
Requires prescription

Commonly Used Brand-Name Products
Capsules, as valproic acid
Depakene 250 mg (also as generic)
Sprinkle capsules
Depakote 125 mg
Tablets, delayed release, as divalproex sodium
Depakote 125 mg, 250 mg, 500 mg
Liquid, as valproate sodium
Depakene and generic as 250 mg/teaspoonful

GENERAL INFORMATION

Very effective in treating bipolar disorder (manic-depressive disorder), especially hard to treat cases, such as rapid cycling. Has also been shown to reduce the number and severity of subsequent episodes of both mania and depression. Valproate can be used alone or in combination with other mood stabilizers in severe cases. It is also used to treat schizoaffective disorder, usually in combination with other medications called antipsychotics.

Before Taking this Medication

Talk to your doctor about the benefits and risks associated with valproate. Make sure you understand how to take it safely and effectively. You and your family members should be very familiar with the side effects and signs of having too much valproate in your system. Make sure your doctor has the following information in detail:

- any allergic or bad reactions you have had to valproate or any other medication
- all prescription and over-the-counter medicines you are taking
- your complete medical history
- if you are pregnant, could be pregnant, or are planning a pregnancy in the near future, valproate should be avoided
- if you are breast-feeding, valproate can pass into breast milk and affect the baby

DOSAGE

The starting dose of valproate will be adjusted based on how you respond and on your blood levels

<u>Adults and adolescents:</u> 500–1500 mg per day, divided in 2 to 4 doses daily.

<u>Older adults</u> are more susceptible to side effects and generally require lower dosages.

<u>Children up to 12:</u> Dosages in this age group are based on body weight.

DIRECTIONS FOR PROPER USE

- *Take exactly as prescribed. Do not take more or less than prescribed. Valproate levels that are too high can cause serious toxicity.*
- If you miss a dose, take it as soon as possible. However, if the missed dose is within 6 hours of your next dose, skip the missed dose and resume with your next scheduled dose. Do not double doses.

- It may take several weeks before you feel the full benefits.
- Laboratory tests are necessary to determine if the amount of valproate in your bloodstream is in the correct range.
- Valproate can cause stomach upset. Taking it with food or meals can lessen this effect. See below for specific directions about the form of valproate you are taking so you can take the necessary precautions.
- <u>If you take the regular capsule form:</u>
  Swallow the capsule whole. Breaking or chewing the capsule can cause irritation of the mouth and throat.
- <u>If you take the long-acting tablet form:</u>
  Swallow the tablet whole. Do not crush, split, or chew it.
  Take with food or meals, but do not take the long-acting tablet form with milk. Milk will cause the special coating to dissolve too soon and cause stomach upset.
  Long-acting tablets are not interchangeable with regular valproate tablets, capsules, or liquid forms.
- <u>If you take the liquid form:</u>
  The liquid form can be mixed with liquids, except carbonated beverages, or added to food, to improve the taste.
- <u>If you take the sprinkle capsule form:</u>
  The capsule contains coated particles of the medicine. The contents of the capsule may be sprinkled over a teaspoonful of semisolid food, such as pudding or applesauce. This mixture should not be chewed. It should not be saved and used at a later time. The sprinkle capsule may also be swallowed whole.

PRECAUTIONS
Alcohol can cause changes in mood and may interfere with valproate's effectiveness. *Alcohol should be avoided while taking valproate.*

Side Effects
Not all side effects will occur. Many side effects will diminish with time. *However, some side effects may be warning signs of toxicity and will require attention from your doctor.* Check with your doctor immediately if you experience any of the following:

- unusual bleeding or bruising, confusion, significant drowsiness, yellow eyes or skin, severe abdominal pain

Some side effects appear when you first start taking valproate and go away for most people. If the following side effects continue, contact your doctor.

- mild hand tremor, mild nausea, mild dizziness, diarrhea or constipation, unusual weight gain or loss, hair loss

Drug Interactions

Valproate can adversely interact with the following frequently prescribed medications:

- anticoagulants (blood thinners)—the effect of the anticoagulant can be increased
- aspirin—when taken in moderate to high doses on a regular basis, can cause increased valproate levels. There is also the possibility of increased bleeding with this combination

MEDICAL CONSIDERATIONS

If you have any of the following medical conditions, make sure your doctor is aware of it.

- liver disease or alcoholism—valproate levels may be higher than expected
- kidney disease—valproate levels may be higher than expected
- anemia or other blood problems—these conditions can be worsened by valproate
- diabetes mellitus (sugar diabetes)—urine ketone levels may be increased

---

Drug Name: VENLAFAXINE   (ven-la-FAX-een)
(serotonin, norepinephrine reuptake inhibitor)

Drug Category: Antidepressant, SNRI
Requires prescription

Commonly Used Brand-Name Products
Tablets
Effexor 25 mg, 37.5 mg, 50 mg, 75 mg, 100 mg
Capsules, extended release
Effexor XR 37.5 mg, 75 mg, 150 mg

GENERAL INFORMATION

Highly effective in treating major depression and the depressed phase of bipolar disorder.

Before Taking this Medication

Talk to your doctor about the benefits and risks associated with venlafaxine. Make sure you understand how to take it safely and effectively. Make sure your doctor has the following information in detail:

- any allergic or bad reactions you have had to venlafaxine or any other medication
- all prescription and over-the-counter medicines you are taking
- your complete medical history
- if you are pregnant, could be pregnant, or are planning a pregnancy in the near future, venlafaxine has not been shown to be absolutely safe
- if you are breast-feeding, venlafaxine can pass into breast milk and affect the baby

DOSAGE

The starting dose of venlafaxine will be low and gradually be increased depending on your response and the side effects you experience.

Adults: 75–350 mg daily.

Older adults are more susceptible to side effects and generally require lower dosages.

Children and adolescents under 18: Safe use in this age group has not been established.

DIRECTIONS FOR PROPER USE

- *Take exactly as prescribed. Do not take more or less than prescribed.*
- Take with food to lessen stomach upset.
- If you miss a dose of the tablet form, take as soon as possible unless it is within 6 hours of your next scheduled dose, then skip the missed dose and resume with your next scheduled dose. Do not double doses.
- It may take several weeks before you feel the full benefits.
- Do not abruptly stop taking venlafaxine unless instructed to do so by your doctor.

PRECAUTIONS

Alcohol can cause changes in mood and may interfere with venlafaxine's effectiveness. *Alcohol should be avoided while taking venlafaxine.*

Side Effects

Not all side effects will occur. Many side effects will diminish with time. *However, some side effects may require attention from your doctor.* Check with your doctor immediately if you experience any of the following:

- increased blood pressure, increased heart rate, skin rash or hives, shortness of breath, chills or fever, swelling of the hands or feet, seizures, sore throat

Some side effects appear when you first start taking venlafaxine and go away for most people. If the following side effects continue, contact your doctor.

- stimulation, anxiety, insomnia, dizziness, sexual problems, sweating, blurred vision, dry mouth, mild to moderate constipation, change in appetite, change in weight, hand tremor, headache

Drug Interactions

Venlafaxine can adversely interact with the following frequently prescribed medications:

- anticoagulants (blood thinners)—the effect of the anticoagulant can be increased
- some nonsedating antihistamines—cardiac (heart) toxicity
- diet pills—severe reaction causing dangerously high blood pressure, high body temperature, seizures, or death
- products containing l-tryptophan—severe reaction causing dangerously high blood pressure, high body temperature, seizures, or death
- cimetidine (Tagamet)—can cause high venlafaxine levels
- TCA antidepressants—can cause high TCA levels
- MAOI antidepressants—severe reaction causing dangerously high blood pressure, high body temperature, seizures, or death
- antipsychotics—may increase certain neurologic side effects
- lithium—increased lithium levels may cause confusion, dizziness, tremor
- anticonvulsants—increased anticonvulsant levels or decreased venlafaxine levels

MEDICAL CONSIDERATIONS

If you have any of the following medical conditions, make sure your doctor is aware of it.

- liver disease or alcoholism—venlafaxine levels may be higher than expected

- kidney disease—venlafaxine levels may be higher than expected
- seizure disorder—venlafaxine can lower seizure threshold
- diabetes mellitus (sugar diabetes)—blood sugar levels may be affected

---

Drug Name: ZOLPIDEM   (ZOLE-pi-dem)

Drug Category: Insomnia medicine
Requires prescription, controlled substance, low potential for abuse

Commonly Used Brand-Name Products
Tablets Ambien 5 mg and 10 mg

GENERAL INFORMATION
Highly effective in treating insomnia.

Before Taking this Medication
Talk to your doctor about the benefits and risks associated with zolpidem. Make sure you understand how to take it safely and effectively. You and your family members should be very familiar with the side effects and signs of having too much zolpidem in your system. Make sure your doctor has the following information in detail:

- any allergic or bad reactions you have had to zolpidem or any other medication
- all prescription and over-the-counter medicines you are taking
- your complete medical history
- if you are pregnant, could be pregnant, or are planning a pregnancy in the near future, zolpidem should not be taken
- if you are breast-feeding, zolpidem can pass into breast milk and affect the baby

DOSAGE
Adults: 5 mg to 10 mg at bedtime.
Older adults are more susceptible to side effects and generally require lower dosages.
Children under 18: Safe use has not been established in this age group.

DIRECTIONS FOR PROPER USE

- *Take exactly as prescribed. Do not take more or less than prescribed. Zolpidem levels that are too high can cause serious toxicity.*
- Zolpidem should **not** be taken with meals, or immediately following meals.
- If you miss a dose, take it as soon as possible if it is within one hour of the scheduled time. However, zolpidem should be taken only if you are sure you will get a full night's sleep of at least 7 to 8 hours.
- If you take zolpidem regularly for an extended period of time, do not stop taking it unless told to do so by your doctor. It may be necessary to gradually reduce the dose before stopping completely.

PRECAUTIONS

Alcohol should be avoided while taking zolpidem.

Side Effects

Not all side effects will occur. Many side effects will diminish with time. *However, some side effects may be warning signs of toxicity and will require attention from your doctor.* Check with your doctor immediately if you experience any of the following:

- confusion, severe drowsiness, slurred speech, severe weakness, unusual thoughts, shortness of breath, excitement, hyperactivity

Some side effects appear when you first start taking zolpidem and go away for most people. If the following side effects continue, contact your doctor.

- dizziness, light-headedness, drowsiness, blurred vision, nausea, diarrhea

Drug Interactions

Significant interactions have not been identified with zolpidem at this time.

MEDICAL CONSIDERATIONS

If you have any of the following medical conditions, make sure your doctor is aware of it.

- liver disease or alcoholism—zolpidem levels may be higher than expected
- kidney disease—zolpidem levels may be higher than expected
- drug dependence or alcohol dependence—the risk for dependence on zolpidem is thought to be low

References

Akiskal, H. S. and R. E. Weise. 1992. The clinical spectrum of so-called "minor" depressions. *American Journal of Psychotherapy* 46: 9–22.

American Psychiatric Association. 1994(a). *Diagnostic and Statistical Manual of Mental Disorders* (Fourth Edition). Washington, D.C.: American Psychiatric Association.

American Psychiatric Association. 1994(b). Practice guidelines for treatment of patients with bipolar disorder. *American Journal of Psychiatry* 151: (Suppl) 1–35.

American Psychiatric Association. 1989. *Treatments of Psychiatric Disorders: A Task Force Report of the American Psychiutric Association.* Washington D. C.: American Psychiatric Association.

American Society of Hospital Pharmacists. 1996. *American Hospital Formulary Service Drug Information.* Bethesda, Md.: American Society of Hospital Pharmacists.

Arndt, S., R. J. Alliger, and N. C. Andreasen. 1991. The distinction of positive and negative symptoms. The failure of a two-dimensional model. *British Journal of Psychiatry* 158: 340–345.

Bachus, S. E. and J. E. Kleinman. 1996. The neuropathology of schizophrenia. The *Journal of Clinical Psychiatry* 57: (Suppl 11) 72–83.

318 Consumer's Guide to Psychiatric Drugs

Ballenger, J. C. and R. M. Post. 1980. Carbamazepine in manic-depressive illness: A new treatment. *American Journal of Psychiatry* 137: 782–790.

Bandura, A. 1991. Self-efficacy mechanism in physiological activation and health promoting behavior. In *Neurobiology of Learning, Emotion and Affect*. Ed. John Madden. New York: Raven Press 229–272.

Baron, M., N. Risch, R. Hamburger, B. Mandel, S. Kushner, M. Newman, D. Drumer, and R. Belmaker. 1987. Genetic linkage between X-chromosome markers and bipolar affective illness. *Nature* 326: 289–292.

Baxter, L. R. 1991. PET studies of cerebral function in major depression and obsessive-compulsive disorder: The emerging profrontal cortex consensus. *Annals of Clinical Psychiatry* 3: 103–109.

Baxter, L. R., J. M. Schwartz, K. S. Bergman, M. P. Szuba, B. H. Guze, J. C. Marriotta, A. Alazvaki, C. E. Selin, H. K. Feung, P. Munford, and M. E. Phelps. 1992. Caudate glucose metabolic rate changes with both drug and behavior therapy for obsessive-compulsive disorder. *Archives of General Psychiatry* 49: 681–689.

Beasley, C. M. and B. E. Dornseif. 1991. Fluoxetine and suicide: A meta-analysis of controlled trials of treatment of depression. *British Medical Journal* 303: 685–692.

Benet, L. Z., J. R. Mitchell, and L. B. Sherner. 1990. General principles. In *Goodman & Gilman's: The Pharmacological Basis of Therapeutics*. Eds. A. G. Gilman, T. W. Rall, A. S. Nies, and P. Taylor. New York: Pergamon Press.

Bloomfield, H., M. Nordfors, and P. McWilliams. 1996. *Hypericum and Depression*. Los Angeles: Prelude Press.

Brotman, A. 1992. *Practical reviews in psychiatry* (audiotape). Birmingham, Ala.: Educational Reviews.

Burton, T. M. 1991. Anti-depression drug of Eli Lilly loses sales after attack by sect. *Wall Street Journal*, April 19, A1–A2.

Calabrese, J. R., S. H. Fatemi, M. Kujawa, and M. J. Woyshville. 1996. Predictors of response to mood stabilizers. *Journal of Clinical Psychopharmacology* 16: (Suppl) 24S–31S.

Castellanos, F. X., J. N. Giedd, P. Eckburg, W. L. Marsh, C. Vaituzis, D. Kaysen, S. D. Hamburger, and J. L. Rapoport. 1994. Quantitative morphology of the caudate nucleus in Attention Deficit Hyperactivity Disorder. *American Journal of Psychiatry* 151: 1791–1796.

Cowley, G., K. Springer, E. A. Leonard, K. Robins and J. Gorden. 1990. The promise of Prozac. *Newsweek* March 26: 38–41.

Davidson, J. R. T. 1997. Atypical depressions. In *Dysthymia and the Spectrum of Chronic Depressions*. Eds. H. S. Akiskal and G. B. Cassano. New York: The Guilford Press. p. 170.

Evans, D. L., M. J. Byerly, and R. A. Greer. 1995. Secondary mania: diagnosis and treatment. *Journal of Clinical Psychiatry* 56: (Suppl) 31–37.

Facts and Comparisons. 1997. St. Louis, Mo.: Facts and Comparisons.

Fava, M. and J. F. Rosenbaum. 1991. Suicidality and fluoxetine: Is there a relationship? *Journal of Clinical Psychiatry* 52: 108–111.

Freud, S. 1940. An Outline of Psychoanalysis. V: *The Standard Edition of the Complete Psychological Works of Sigmund Freud*. Vol. 23:141–208. London: Hogarth Press.

Gerber, P. D., J. Barrett, E. Manheimer, R. Whiting, and R. Smith. 1989. Recognition of depression by internists in primary care. *Journal of General Internal Medicine*, 4: 7–13.

Goldberg, J. F., M. Harrow, and L. S. Grossman. 1995. Course and outcome in bipolar affective disorder: A longitudinal follow-up study. *American Journal of Psychiatry* 152: 379–384.

Gordon, B. 1990. *I'm Dancing as Fast as I Can*. New York: Bantam.

Gunderson, J. G. 1984. *Borderline Personality Disorder*. Washington, D.C.: American Psychiatric Press.

Hamilton, Max. 1989. Mood disorders: Clinical features. In *Comprehension Textbook of Psychiatry*. Eds. H. I. Kaplan and B. J. Sadock. Baltimore: Williams and Wilkins. p. 897.

Hartocollis, P., Ed. 1977. *Borderline Personality Disorders*. New York: International Universities Press.

Hill, J. C. and E. P. Schoener. 1994. Age-dependent decline of attention deficit hyperactivity disorder. *American Journal of Psychiatry* 153: 1143–1146.

Hollister, L. E., B. Muller-Oerlinghausen, K. Rickels and R. I. Shader. 1993. Clinical uses of benzodiazepines. *Journal of Clinical Psychopharmacology* 13: (Suppl 1) 1S–150S.

Jaskiw, G. E. and D. R. Weinberger. 1992. Dopamine and schizophrenia—a cortically corrective perspective. *Seminars in the Neurosciences* 4: 179–188.

Jencks, S. F. 1985. Recognition of mental distress and diagnosis of mental disorder in primary care. *JAMA* 253: 1903–1907.

Judd, L. L., D. L. Braff, K. T. Britton, S. C. Risch, J. C. Gillin, and I. Grant. Psychiatry and medicine. 1991. In *Harris's Principles of Internal Medicine*. Eds. J. D. Wilson, E. Braunwald, K. J. Isselbacher, R. G. Petersdorf, J. B. Martin, A. S. Fauci and R. K. Root. New York: McGraw-Hill.

Keck, P. E. and S. L. McElroy. 1996. Outcome in the pharmacologic treatment of bipolar disorder. *Journal of Clinical Psychopharmacology* 16: (Suppl) 15S–23S.

Keller, M. B., P. Lavori, W. Coryell, J. Endicott, and T. I. Mueller. 1993. Bipolar I: A five-year prospective follow-up. *Journal of Nervous and Mental Disease* 181: 238–245.

Kessler, R. C., K. A. McGonagle, S. Zhao, C. B. Nelson, M. Hughes, S. Eshleman, H. Wittchen, and K. S. Kendler. 1994. Lifetime and 12-month prevalence of DSM-III-R psychiatric disorders in the United States. *Archives of General Psychiatry* 51: 8–19.

Kramer, P. D. 1993. *Listening to Prozac*. New York: Viking.

Kreisman, J. J. and H. Strauss. 1989. *I Hate You, Don't Leave Me: Understanding the Borderline Personality*. New York: Avon Books.

Linehan, M. M. 1993. *Cognitive Behavioral Treatment of Borderline Personality Disorder*. New York: Guilford Press.

Lydiard, R. B. and S. A. Falsetti. 1995. Treatment options for social phobia. *Psychiatric Annals* 25: 570–576.

Mahler, M. S., F. Pine, and A. Bergman. 1975. *The Psychological Birth of the Human Infant*. New York: Basic Books.

National Institute of Mental Health. D/ART. 1990. Fact Sheet.

Nies, A. S. 1990. Principles of therapeutics. In *Goodman & Goodman's: The Pharmacological Basis of Therapeutics*. Eds. A. G. Gilman, T. W. Rall, A. S. Nies and P. Taylor. New York: Pergamon Press.

Norden, M. J. 1995. *Beyond Prozac.* New York: HarperCollins.

Norden, M. J. 1989(a). Fluoxetine in borderline personality disorder. *Progress in Neuropsychopharmacological Biological Psychiatry,* 13: 885–893.

Norden, M. J. 1989(b). Is there an effective drug treatment for borderline personality disorder? *Harvard Mental Health Letter* 6: 8.

Ornstein, R. and R. F. Thompson. 1984. *The Amazing Brain.* Boston: Houghton Mifflin.

Perez-Stable, E. J., J. Miranda, R. F. Munoz, Y. Ying. 1990. Depression in medical outpatients: under-recognition and misdiagnosis. *Archives of Internal Medicine* 150: 1083–1088.

Preston, J. D., J. H. O' Neal, and M.C. Talaga. 1997. *Handbook of Clinical Psychopharmacology for Therapists.* Second Edition. Oakland, CA: New Harbinger Publications.

Preston, J. D. 1997. *Shorter-Term Treatment for Borderline Personality Disorders.* Oakland, CA: New Harbinger Publications.

Redmond, D. E., Jr. 1985. Neurochemical basis for anxiety and anxiety disorders: evidence from drugs which decrease human fear or anxiety. In *Anxiety and Anxiety Disorders.* Eds. A. H. Tuma and J. D. Maser. NJ: Hillsdale. 533–555.

Rosenthal, N. E. 1994. Seasonal Affective Disorder: Update. Presentation delivered at the 1994 NIMH, D/ART annual meeting, Rockville, MD.

Roth, M. 1996. The Panic-Agoraphobic Syndrome: A paradigm of the anxiety group of disorders and its implications for psychiatric practice and theory. *American Journal of Psychiatry* 153: (Suppl) 111–124.

Safer, D. J. and J. M. Krager. 1992. Effect of a media blitz and a threatened lawsuit on stimulant treatment. *JAMA* 268: 1004–1007.

Schwartz, J. M. 1996. *Brainlock.* New York: Reganbooks.

Silver, D. and M. Rosenbluth. Eds. 1992. *Handbook of Borderline Disorders.* Madison, CT: International Universities Press.

Solomon, D. A., G. J. Keitner, J. W. Miller, M. T. Shea, and M. B. Keller. 1995. Course of illness and maintenance treatments for patients with bipolar disorder. *Journal of Clinical Psychiatry* 56: 5–13.

Stewart, J. W., F. J. Quitkin, and D. F. Klein. 1992. The pharmacotherapy of minor depression. *American Journal of Psychotherapy* 46: 23–36.

Susann, J. 1997. *Once Is Not Enough.* New York: Grove Atlantic.

Teicher, M. H., C. Glod, and J. O. Cole. 1990. Emergence of intense suicidal preoccupation during fluoxetine treatment. *American Journal of Psychiatry* 147: 207-210.

Tsuang, M. T. and S. V. Faraone. 1990. *The Genetics of Mood Disorders.* Baltimore: John Hopkins University Press.

Weinberger, D. R. 1996. On the plausibility of "the neurodevelopmental hypothesis" of schizophrenia. *Neuropsychopharmacology* 14: 15–115.

Zametkin, A. J., T. E. Nordahl, M. Gross, A. C. King, W. E. Semple, J. Rumsey, S. D. Hamburger, and R. M. Cohen. 1990. Cerebral glucose metabolism in adults with hyperactivity of childhood onset. *New England Journal of Medicine* 323: 1361–1366.

Zisook, S. 1996. Bereavement: Grief, Depression, Anxiety. *Audio Digest Psychiatry* (audiotape). Glendale, CA: Audio Digest Foundation.

Recommended Reading

Andreason, N. 1995. *The Broken Brain: The Biological Revolution in Psychiatry*. New York: HarperCollins.

Briggs, G. G. 1992. Drugs in pregnancy and lactation. In *Applied Therapeutics: The Clinical Use of Drugs*. Fifth Edition. M. A. Koda-Kimble, L. Y. Young, W. A. Kradjan, and B. J. Guglielmo. Eds. Vancouver, Wash.: Applied Therapeutics.

Brown, C. S. and S. G. Bryant. 1992. Major depressive disorders. In *Applied Therapeutics: The Clinical Use of Drugs*. Fifth Edition. M. A. Koda-Kimble, L. Y. Young, W. A. Kradjan, and B. J. Guglielmo. Eds. Vancouver, Wash.: Applied Therapeutics.

Burns, David. 1980. *Feeling Good*. New York: New American Library.

Cornelius, J. R., P. H. Soloff, J. M. Perel, and R. F. Ulrich. 1991. A preliminary trial of fluoxetine in refractory borderline patients. *Journal of Clinical Psychopharmacology* 11: 116–120.

Cowdry, R. W. and D. L. Gardner. 1988. Pharmacotherapy of borderline personality disorder. *Archives of General Psychiatry* 45: 111–119.

Davidson, J., H. Kudler, R. Smith, S. L. Mahoney, S. Lipper, E. Hammett, W. B. Saunders, and J. O. Cavenar. 1990. Treatment of PTSD with amitriptyline and placebo. *Archives of General Psychiatry* 47: 259–266.

Davidson, J., S. Roth, and E. Newman. 1991. Fluoxetine in post-traumatic stress disorder. *Journal of Traumatic Stress* 4: 419–423.

Davis, K., R. Kahn, G. Ko, and M. Davidson. 1991. Dopamine in schizophrenia: A review and reconceptualization. *American Journal of Psychiatry* 148: 1474–1484.

Ereshefsky, L. and A. L. Richards. 1992. Psychoses. In *Applied Therapeutics: The Clinical Use of Drugs*. Fifth Edition. M. A. Koda-Kimble, L. Y. Young, W. A. Kradjan, B. J. Guglielmo. Eds. Vancouver: Wash.: Applied Therapeutics.

Fava, M., K. I. Anderson, and J. Rosenbaum. 1993. Are thynoleptic responsive anger attacks a discrete clinical syndrome? *Psychosouratics* 34(4).

Frances, A. J. 1989. *Borderline Personality Disorder* (audiotape). New York: Guilford Publications.

Frances, A. J. and P. H. Soloff, 1998. Treating the borderline patient with low-dose neuroleptics. *Hospital and Community Psychiatry* 39: 246–248.

George, A. and P. H. Soloff. 1986. Schizotypal symptoms in patients with borderline personality disorder. *American Journal of Psychiatry* 143: 212–215.

Goldberg, S. C., S. C. Schulz, P. M. Schulz, R. J. Resnick, R. M. Hamer, and R. O. Friedel. 1986. Borderline and schizotypal personality disorders treated with low-dose thiothixene vs. placebo. *Archives of General Psychiatry* 43: 680–686.

Hunt, R. D. 1997. Nosology, neurobiology, and clinical patterns of ADHD in adults. *Psychiatric Annals* 27: 572–581.

Javitt, D. and S. Zukin. 1991. Recent advances in the phencyclidine model of schizophrenia. *American Journal of Psychiatry* 148: 1301–1307.

Kety, S. S. 1975. Progress toward an understanding of the biological substrates of schizophrenia. In *Genetic Research in Psychiatry*. R. R. Fieve, et al. Eds. Baltimore: Johns Hopkins University Press.

Kety, S. S., D. Rosenthal, T. H. Wender, and F. Schulsinger. 1971. Mental illness in the biological and adoptive families of adopted schizophrenics. *American Journal of Psychiatry* 128: 302–306.

Liebowitz, M. R. and D. F. Klein. 1981. Interrelationships of hysteroid-dysphoria and borderline personality disorder. *Psychiatric Clinics of North America*, 4: 67–87.

Luby, E. D., J. S. Gottlieb, B. D. Cohen, G. Rosenbaum, and E. F. Domino. 1962. Model psychoses and schizophrenia. *American Journal of Psychiatry* 119: 61–67.

Luby, E. D., M. A. Marrazzi, and J. Kinzie. 1987. Letter to the editor. *Journal of Clinical Psychopharmacology* 7: 52–53.

Malaspina, O., H. M. Quitkin, and C. A. Kaufmann. 1992. Epidemiology and genetics of neuropsychiatric disorders. In *The American Psychiatric Press Textbook of Neuropsychiatry* S. C. Yudofsky and R. E. Hales. Eds. Washington, D. C.: American Psychiatric Press.

Markovitz, P. J., J. R. Calabrese, S. C. Schulz, et al. 1991. Fluoxetine in the treatment of borderline and schizotypal personality disorders. *American Journal of Psychiatry* 148: 1064–1067.

Meyer, U. A. 1992. Drugs in special patient groups: Clinical importance of genetics in drug effects. In *Melmon and Morrelli's Clinical Pharmacology: Basic Principles in Therapeutics*. Third Edition. K. L. Melmon, H. F. Morrelli, B. B. Hoffman, and D. W. Nierenberg. Eds. New York: McGraw-Hill.

Nagy, L. M., C. A. Morgan, S. M. Southwick, and D. S. Charney. 1993. Open prospective trial of fluoxetine for post-traumatic stress disorder. *Journal of Clinical Psychopharmacology* 13: 107–113.

Preston, John. 1996. *You Can Beat Depression*. Second Edition. San Luis Obispo, CA: Impact Publishers.

Rubin, P. C. 1992. Drugs in special patient groups: Pregnancy and nursing. In *Melmon and Morrelli's Clinical Pharmacology: Basic Principles in Therapeutics*. Third Edition. K. L. Melmon, H. F. Morrelli, B. B. Hoffman, and D. W. Nierenberg. Eds. New York: McGraw-Hill.

Salzman, C., A. N. Wolfson, A. Schatzberg, et al. 1995. Effect of fluoxetine on anger in symptomatic volunteers with borderline personality disorder. *Journal of Clinical Psychopharmacology* 15(1): 23–29.

Smith, D. E. and D. R. Wesson. 1983. Benzodiazepine dependency syndromes. *Journal of Psychoactive Drugs* 15: 85–95.

Snodgrass, W. R. 1992. Drugs in special patient groups: Neonates and children. In *Melmon and Morrelli's Clinical Pharmacology: Basic Principles in Therapeutics*. Third Edition. K. L. Melmon, H. F. Morrelli, B. B. Hoffman, and D. W. Nierenberg. Eds. New York: McGraw-Hill.

Soloff, P. H., A. George, R. S. Nathan, P. M. Schulz, R. F. Ulrich, and J. M. Perel. 1986. Progress in psychopharmacology of borderline disorders. *Archives of General Psychiatry* 43: 691–697.

Stone, M. H. 1988. Toward a psychobiological theory of borderline disorder. *Dissociation* 1: 2–15.

Torrey, E. F. 1983. *Surviving Schizophrenia: A Family Manual*. New York: Harper and Row.

Ulenhuth, E. H., H. DeWit, M. B. Balter, C. E. Johanson, and G. D. Mellinger. 1988. Risks and benefits of long term benzodiazepine use. *Journal of Clinical Psychopharmacology* 8: 161–167.

van der Kolk, B. A. 1987. *Psychological Trauma*. Washington, D. C.: American Psychiatric Press.

Vestal, R. E., S. C. Montamat, and C. P. Nielson. 1992. Drugs in special patient groups: The elderly. In *Melmon and Morrelli's Clinical Pharmacology: Basic Principles in Therapeutics*. Third Edition. K. L. Melmon, H. F. Morrelli, B. B. Hoffman, and D. W. Nierenberg. Eds. New York: McGraw-Hill.

Weinberger, D. R., K. F. Berman, R. Suddath, and E. F. Torrey. 1992. Evidence of dysfunction of a prefrontal-limbic network in schizophrenia: A magnetic resonance imaging and regional cerebral blood flow study of discordant monozygotic twins. *American Journal of Psychiatry* 149: 890–897.

Winchel, R. M. and M. Stanley. 1991. Self-injurious behavior: A review of the behavior and biology of self-mutilation. *American Journal of Psychiatry* 148: 306–317.

Resources

Alzheimer's Disease and Related Disorders Association.
919 North Michigan Avenue
Suite 1000
Chicago, IL 60611
312-335-8700
(This is a national organization for caregivers.)

National Alliance for the Mentally Ill (NAMI)
200 N. Glebe Rd., Suite 1015
Arlington, VA 22203-3754
703-524-7600 Fax 703-524-9094
Help Line 1-800-950-6264
Website www.nami.org

The National Depressive and Manic-Depressive Association
1-800-826-3632

National Institute of Mental Health, Depression Awareness Program 1-800-421-4211

National Mental Health Association, Campaign on Clinical Depression 1-800-969-NMHA

Obsessive-Compulsive Foundation
P. O. Box 70
Milford, CT 06460-0070
203-878-5669

Index

Abandonment, 136
Abuse, substance
    and aggression, 140
    and anxiety disorders, 103-104,
        110–111, 114
    and attention deficit disorder, 134
    and bipolar disorders, 82, 84, 99,
        103
    and depression, 49–50
    family history of, 99, 109, 134
    and post-traumatic stress disor-
        der, 139
    prevalence of, 8, 15
    and psychosis, 120
    See also Addiction; Alcohol
Adapin, 65, 209
Addiction, 2, 15
    and anorexia, 134
    antidepressants and antipsychot-
        ics as nonaddictive medica-
        tions, 23, 71, 109, 127
    awareness of potential for, 17, 99,
        104, 107
    and dependency, differences be-
        tween, 108–110, 113
    and major depression, 50
    and psychotropic medications, 23,
        71, 74, 99, 106–109, 112, 132
    and post-traumatic stress disor-
        der, 138, 140
    See also Abuse, substance; Alco-
        hol
Adjuncts and alternatives to treatment
    of psychological disorders, 153–160
Adolescents. See Children
Age and medication treatment, 4,
    67–68, 95, 145, 147–151
    See also Children; Elderly

Aggression and disorders associated
    with increase in serotonin, 84,
    140–141, 157
Agoraphobia and panic, 112
Agranulocytosis, 126
Akathesia side effects, 125–126
Akineton, 123
Alcohol
    and aggression, 140
    and anxiety disorders, 103–104,
        110, 114
    dementia, 141
    and depression, 50, 56–59, 61, 71,
        75
    as interfering with nerve cell
        function, 33–35
    and drug interaction dangers, 2,
        62–63, 71, 98–99, 104, 160
    and mania, 84
    and sleep patterns, 155
    withdrawal and psychosis, 120
Aldomet, 56
Allergies and medication, 70–71, 126
Alprazolam, 105, 166–168
Altarax, 105, 107–108, 177
Alzheimer's disease
    as cause of psychosis, 117, 121
    treatment for, 141–142
Amantadine, 56, 123, 176
Amantadine hydrochloride, 56
Ambien, 105, 314
American Psychiatric Association,
    81–82, 85–88, 117–118, 141
American Society of Hospital Pharma-
    cists, 145
Amitriptyline, 65, 168–171
Amoxapine, 65, 171–173
Amphetamine, 173–176

Anafranil, 193
Angina pectoris and anxiety, 103
Anhedonia
    and depression, 35, 52–54, 84–85
    and schizophrenia, 119
Anphetamine, 63, 173
Antianxiety medication
    addiction and dependency poten-
        tial, 109
    with antipsychotic medication,
        128
    and anxiety disorders, 104–115
    and attention deficit disorder, 133
    and bipolar disorders, 90
    and borderline personality disor-
        der, 137
    and dementia, 142
    and depression, 56–57, 74
    and psychotic disorders, 127
    types and dosages, 105–106, 114
Anticholinergic side effects
    and antipsychotic medication, 86,
        123, 126
    and antidepressant medication,
        65
Anticholinergics, 176–177
Anticonvulsant medication
    and aggression, 140–141
    and attention deficit disorder, 133
    and bipolar disorder, 87–88,
        90–91, 95–98
    and pregnancy and breastfeeding,
        146
Antidepressant medication
    and antipsychotic medication, 79,
        129
    and anxiety disorders, 110–111,
        113–114, 116
    and attention deficit disorder,
        133–134
    biological interferences with, 64,
        66
    and borderline personality disor-
        ders, 137
    cautions and contraindications of,
        70–71
    and children, 16, 147–148
    classes of
        MAO inhibitors, 62–3, 65,
            110–111, 146
        standard, 62, 64–65, 71
    and dementia, 142
    duration of treatment, 72–73, 113
    effect on nerve cells, 59–61
    expectations from, 66–70
    ineffectiveness of when combined
        with mood stabilizers for bi-
        polar disorders, 90
    as not addictive nor habit-
        forming, 71, 74, 109

    and pregnancy breastfeeding,
        144–146
    side effects, 23, 66, 70, 113
    treatment phases in using, 68–70
    as trigger for manic episode, 86,
        98
Antidyskinetics, 176–177
Antihistamines, 63, 107–108, 177–178
Antihypertensives as cause of depres-
    sion, 56
Antiparkinsonian medication, 57,
    124–126
Antipsychotic medication
    and aggression, 140–141
    and awareness of drug distribu-
        tion within body, 41–42
    and bipolar disorders, 90
    and effect of pregnancy and
        newborn, 146
    growth of, 11, 26–27
    as not addictive nor habit-
        forming, 127
    and psychotic disorders, 121–128
Anxiety disorders
    and antidepressant medication,
        74
    and attention deficit disorder, 131
    and atypical depression, 78
    case histories, 12–14, 33–34
    degree, prevalence, and severity
        of, 2–3, 7–9, 20
    and environmental factors be-
        hind, 33–34
    medical causes of, 102–103
    types and treatment, 101-115
    See also Symptoms; Treatment
Apathy and depression, 54, 59, 84
Apresoline hydrochloride, 56
Aricept, 141
Artane, 123, 176
Asendin, 65, 171
Atarax, 105, 107
Atenolol, 105, 110, 178
Ativan, 105, 236
Attention deficit disorder (ADD)
    and function within brain, 30,
        131–132
    treatment of, 16, 132–134, 147
Attention deficit disorder/hyperactiv-
    ity disorder (ADHD), 131
Atypical antipsychotics
    as alternative in bipolar disorder
        treatment, 100
    as psychosis treatment, 121, 124
Atypical depression, 78
Atypical psychosis, 117, 119
Augmentation strategies in treatment,
    73, 99–100
Aventyl, 65, 256
Awareness

of diagnosis and of treatment
available, 1–2
of drug processes within body,
41–42
Benadryl, 105, 177
Benefits of medication, 43–46
Benzedrine, 63
Benzodiazepines, 146
Benztropine, 86, 123, 176
Benztropine mesylate, 123
Beta-blockers, 178–179
and aggression, 140–141
as anxiety disorders treatment,
107–108, 110, 113, 115
Bioavailability, 40–41
Biological changes and treatment outcome, 61
Biological disturbances as interfering
with antidepressant medication, 64,
66
Biological rhythms as monitoring
sleep patterns and energy levels,
29, 87
Biology of disorders, understanding
of, 4, 10, 27–36, 55, 87
Biotransformation, 40, 42–43
Bipolar disorders
and aggression, 140
physiological, genetic, and environmental causes of, 87–88
caution in use of light therapy
treatment for, 76
characteristics and symptoms of,
81–85
medication for, development and
expectations of, 23, 27, 90–98
hypomania, 83, 85–86, 98
subtypes, 85–86
See also Depression; Drugs; Mania
Bipolar I, II, characteristics of, 85–86
Birth control pills and depression,
56–57
Biperiden, 123
Blood and effects of anticonvulsant
medication, 95, 97
Blood pressure
and antihypertensive medication,
56
and antipsychotic medication,
126
and beta blockers, 108, 110
and the elderly, 150
medication and drug-drug intera-
tions, 63, 86
Borderline personality disorders,
135–138
Brain
and anxiety disorders, 112,
114–116
and bipolar disorders, 87–90

chemistry and interference with
normal functioning, 33
and depression, 59–63
and eating disorders, 134–135
and effects of sleep deprivation,
154
of fetus and effects of medication
on, 144–146
injury, trauma, and tumors as associated with mania, 86
and positive effects antidepressant medication on neuro-
transmitters serotonin,
dopamine, and norepineph-
rine, 60-63
and psychosis, 117, 119–121
structure of, 28–36
technological developments and
understanding of, 10, 38–39,
115, 121
Brain centers
hypothalamus and limbic system,
28–30, 59
and pleasure activated by neurochemicals, 34–35
Brand names of drugs directory,
163–165
Breast feeding and effects of medication, 145–146
Bromocriptine, 130
Bulimia, 134–135
Bupropion, 65, 98, 135, 146, 179–182
Bupropion–S.R., 65
BuSpar, 63, 105, 182
Buspirone, 63, 105, 113, 114–116,
140–141, 182–184
Caffeine and anxiety, 103, 113
Calcium channel blockers as alternative or addition to treatment, 100
Carbamazepine, 90–91, 94–95, 141,
146, 184–187
Cardiac arrhythmia and anxiety, 103
Case histories and diagnoses, 12–14,
33–34
Catapres, 56, 105, 197
Cautions and warnings in treatment,
161–162
Cautions and contraindications
and alcohol, 58, 71
with antidepressant medications,
68, 70–71, 135
with antianxiety medications,
97–100, 106–107
driving and drugs, 161–162
of light therapy for bipolar disorder treatment, 76
in prescribing medication for borderline personality disorders,
137
with stimulants, 133–134

and storage of medications, 162
Centrax, 105
Cerebral degenerative disease and
   psychosis, 121
Chemical
   activity within brain, 29–32,
      34–35, 62, 77–78
   alteration of and psychiatric
      symptoms, 27–28, 53–55, 115,
      132, 155
   blood-brain barrier to limit inges-
      tion of drug toxins, 40–41
   differences in antidepressant
      makeup, 62–67
   estrogen, 77–78
Chemical straitjacket and history of
   drug development, 11, 14
Childbirth and bipolar disorders, 85
Children
   attention deficit disorder and at-
      tention deficit/hyperactivity
      disorder (ADHD) in, 15–16,
      131–134
   and borderline personality disor-
      der, 136–137
   and drug intake during preg-
      nancy, 97–98, 143–147
   and Ritalin, 15–16, 132–133
   See also Safety
Chlordiazepoxide, 56, 105, 187–189
Chlorpromazine, 122–123, 189–192
Chronic neurobiological malfunction,
   77
Church of Scientology and negative
   publicity, 15–16
Cibalith, Cibalith-S, 92, 232
Circadian cycle, 87
Clinical depression. *See* Depression
Clinical social workers, 20, 60
Clomipramine, 116, 192–195
Clonazepam, 105, 130, 195–197
Clonidine, 105, 133, 140–141, 197–198
Clonidine hydrochloride, 56
Clorazepate, 105, 198–201
Clozapine, 100, 122, 126, 201–203
Clozaril, 122, 201
Cocaine, 63, 74
Cogentin, 123, 176
Cognex, 141
Cognitive behavioral therapy
   for anxiety disorders treatment,
      14, 112–113, 115–116
   and depression, 9, 50, 60
   See also Psychotherapy
Complicated grief and potential for
   major depression, 52
Concentration, impairment of as
   symptom of depression and atten-
   tion deficit disorder, 30, 54, 84
Control

of alcohol intake and depression,
   58
of emotions and chemical brain
   activity, 29–30, 111, 135, 140,
   156
regaining as result of medication,
   68
regaining as result of psychother-
   apy, 36, 140
Core symptoms. *See* Symptoms
Corgard, 178
Cortex, function and parts of, 30–31,
   121, 132
Corticosteroids and depression, 57
Cortisone acetate, 57
Cortone, 57
Cosmetic psychopharmacology, 23
Counselors, licensed, 21
CT (computerized tomography) 27–28
Cyclic patterns of bipolar disorder,
   characteristics of, 81–82, 85–87
Cyclothymia as subtype of mania,
   85–86
Cylert, 266
Dalmane, 105, 219
Decongestant, avoidance of when
   prone to panic attacks, 103, 113
Delusions and schizophrenia, 117,
   119–120
Dementia and psychotic disorders,
   117, 120–121, 141–142
Demerol, 63
Depakote, 95–96, 308
Depakene, 95–96, 308
Dependency verses addiction,
   108–109, 111
Depo-Provera, 57
Depression
   and anxiety, 13–14, 110, 114
   and attention deficit disorder, 131
   awareness of severity of, 20
   and bulimia, 135
   and cyclic patterns in bipolar dis-
      orders, 85–87
   drugs and medical disorders as
      trigger of, 55–58, 110, 114
   dysthymia and premenstrual dys-
      phoria, 76–78
   and the elderly, 149–150
   and genetics, 55
   major, or clinical
      diagnosis, characteristics, and
         symptoms of, 38, 51–5,
         59, 61, 84–85
      atypical and psychotic as sub-
         types of, 78–79, 118
   and malfunctions of cortex, 31,
      35
   medication side effects as cause
      of, 32

melatonin and St. John's Wort
for, 159–160
and positive personality change
after medication treatment
program, 23–24
and Prozac, negative publicity,
16–17, 23
and serotonin, methods to increase, 155–158
success in psychotherapy treatment for, 9, 50, 60
treatment for, 59–80
understanding of and medical
approach to relief from, 2–4,
9, 14, 19
See also Antidepressant medication; Bipolar disorders; Treatment
Desipramine, 65, 203–206
Desyrel, 65, 298
Dexedrine, 63, 71, 74, 132–133, 174
Dextroamphetamine, 174
Dextromethorphan, 63
Diagnosis
of anxiety disorders, 109–112,
114–115
of attention deficit disorder, 131
of bipolar disorders, 82–84, 99
of borderline personality disorder, 136
of dementia, 141
of depression, 51–57, 73
of psychotic disorders, 78–79,
109, 118–120, 128
of post-traumatic stress disorder,
138–139
of sleep disorders, 129–130
See also Schizophernia
Diagnostic and Statistical Manual of
Mental Disorders (DSM–IV), 136
Diazepam, 56, 105, 206–209
Diet
and depression, 56, 59, 75, 78, 84
as healthy to regulate neurotransmitters, 157–160
and MAO-inhibitors antidepressant medication, foods to
avoid, 62–63
Diphenhydramine, 105, 177
Directory, brand names, 163–165
Disorders, medical. *See* Medical disorders
Disorders, psychological
nerve cells involved, 32–33
types and prevalence of, 7–8, 38
See also specific name of disorder
Disorganized thinking
and antipsychotic medication, 121
and borderline personality disor-

der, 137
and depression, 3, 79
and mania, 83
and schizophrenia, 31, 117, 119
Diurnal variations in mood as symptom of depression, 84
Divalproex sodium, 96
Doctor-patient cooperation in medication management, 39, 43–44, 46–47,
57, 63, 66–67, 74, 92–93, 96, 98,
100, 126, 144, 147–149, 159
Donepezil, 141
Dopamine, as neurotransmitting nerve
cell and chemical affected in psychological disorders, 31–35, 59–61,
64, 87–88, 121, 130
Doral, 105, 278
Doxepin,65, 209–212
Dramatization as symptom of mania,
83
Drug tables, charts, and directory,
56–57, 65, 92, 105, 109, 122–123,
141, 146, 163–165
Drugs
anticonvulsants, 90–99
antipsychotics, 11, 26–27, 121–128
basis processes of within body,
39–43
as cause psychological disorders,
56–57, 86–87,102–103, 110
and children and adolescents,
145–148
dangers of drug–drug interactions, 2, 22, 33–34, 62–63, 67,
77, 91, 98, 103–104, 106, 149,
159–160
defined, 39
dependency and addiction potential, 104, 106, 108–112, 114,
132–133
dosage
monitoring of, 44–47, 65,
67–68, 73, 89–92, 94,
96–98,105, 107, 113,
122–128, 149, 151
and regularity in taking, 67,
89, 148
and long-term use, 69–74, 127,
132–134
and pregnancy and breastfeeding,
70–71, 97–98, 143
and sleep disorders, 130
storage of, 162
See also Addiction; Management
of medications; Safety
Duper, 57
Dystonia side effect, 125
Dysthymia as low-grade and long-
lasting depression type, 76–77

Dysregulation in neurotransmitter system as characteristic of psychological disorders, 59, 87, 112

Eating disorders, 134–135

Education and lifestyle changes necessary to minimize bipolar disorder episodes, 88–90

Effexor, 65, 311

Effexor XR, 311

Elavil, 65, 168

Elderly and medication treatment, 149–151

Electro-convulsive therapy (ECT), 79–80, 100

Elector-encephalogram (EEG), 130

Electrolyte imbalance and psychosis, 120

Emotional paralysis and major depression, 50–51, 54, 68

Empowerment and awareness of treatment alternatives, 22–23

Emptiness, 53, 119, 136

Endorphins, 34–35, 134–135

Endrocinopathy and psychosis, 120

Epilepsy and psychosis, 120

Eskalith, 65, 92, 232

Eskalith CR, 232

Estazolam, 105, 212–214

Estraderm, 57

Estrace, 57

Estrogen, 57, 77

Euphorism as symptom of mania, 83, 85, 118

Evaluation
  of effectiveness of medications, 68, 73–74, 90–91, 104
  of medical diagnosis, necessity of, 4, 13, 33, 58, 87, 103, 141

Evavil, 168

Excretion as a process of drug distribution within body, 40, 43

Exercise, 75, 113, 134, 154, 156–157

Expectations of medication treatment, 66–70, 91–92, 94–96, 104, 106–107, 132–133

Extropyramidal side effects, types of, 122, 125–126

Family
  children and psychotropic medication, 145, 147–148
  and education on medication, 17
  and bipolar disorders
    genetics of, 88
    impact of patient's behavior on, 82
  history for accurate diagnosis of depression, 55, 57, 99
  and schizophrenia, 120
  support from, 57

Fatigue, 20, 29, 56, 59, 68, 76–77, 84, 93, 95, 114, 133, 154
  See also Sleep

Federal Drug Administration (FDA), 16, 159

Fight or flight response in anxiety, 101–102, 104, 114

Flight of ideas as symptom of mania, 83

Fluphenazine, 123, 217–219

Flurazepam, 105, 219–221

Fluoxetine, 65, 113, 116, 135, 214–216

Fluvoxamine, 65, 221–224

Foods, chemical makeup of and negative interactions with MAO-inhibitor antidepressants, 62–63

Functionality, impairment of, 50–53, 82–83

Gabapentin, 90–91, 97

Gamma-amino butyric acid (GABA), 33, 87–88, 95–96, 106

Gene mapping, 28

Generalized anxiety disorder
  cognitive–behavioral therapy for, 115
  diagnosis and medical treatment for, 114–115
  as type of anxiety disorder, 102

Genetics as factor in psychiatric disorders, 33, 55, 87–88, 132, 134, 147

Ginseng, 74

Glaucoma and antidepressants, 70–71

Glutamate as implicated in psychiatric disorders, 32–33

Goals of psychiatric treatment, 14, 34

Grandiosity as symptom of mania, 83

Grief verses major depression, 51–53

Group therapy. *See* Psychotherapy

Guanelhidine sulfate, 56

Hair loss and anticonvulsant medication, 97

Halazepam, 224–226

Halcion, 105, 301

Haldol, 123, 226

Haldol decanoate, 226

Half-life defined, 43

Hallucinations
  and antipsychotic medication for, 121–123
  and mania, 83
  and psychotic disorders, 79, 117–120

Haloperidol, 122–124, 226–229

Hormone imbalances
  and antipsychotic medication, 126
  as cause of psychosis, 117, 120
  light therapy for, 75–76
  and premenstrual dysphoria, 77

Health
  effects of depression on, 50

foods, herbs, and mood disorders, 158–160
Heart
    attack and antidepressant medication, 70
    and anticonvulsant medication on, 95
History
    and improvements in limiting side effects of medications, 62
    medical, necessary in drug treatment program, 43–44, 66, 99, 103, 109, 114, 134, 149
    of psychological disorders and treatment for, 8–11, 25–27, 37, 74, 121
    medical and technological advances to understanding psychiatric conditions, 37–38, 51, 62, 121
Hopelessness, 81
Hospitalization, 83, 89, 123–124
Huntington's chorea and psychosis, 121
Hydralazine hydrochloride, 56
Hydroxyzine, 105, 107–108, 115, 177
Hyperthyroidism, 86, 102–103, 120
Hypoglycemia and psychosis, 120
Hypomania, 83, 85, 98
    See also Bipolar disorder; Mania
Hypothalamus
    dysfunction and depression, 59
    functions of, 28–30
Hypothyroidism and depression, 50, 94
Hypoxia and psychosis, 120
Illness, physical, and depression, 50
Imipramine, 65, 72, 113, 229–232
Immune system, impact of depression on, 50
Impulsiveness, 136
Inderal, 56, 105, 178
Infections as cause of disorders, 56, 86, 120
Insomnia, 29, 33, 54–55. *See also* Sleep
Interpersonal therapy, 60
Irritability
    and increase in serotonin, 154, 157
    as symptom of depression and mania, 54, 83–85
Ismelin sulfate, 56
Judgment, impairment of as symptom of psychotic depression and mania, 79, 84
Kindling, 87–88, 94
Kidney
    and anticonvulsant medication, 93–94
    failure and psychosis, 120

Klonopin, 105, 195
Laboratory tests
    accurate diagnosis of anxiety disorder dependent on, 103
    frequency necessary with anticonvulsants and mood stabilizers, 87, 92, 95, 126
    and schizophrenia, 120
Lamectal, 97
Lamotrigine, 90–91, 97
Legal requirements for prescriptions, 148
Levodapa, 57, 63
Levodapa carbidopa, 57
Levothyroxine as inducing mania, 86
Librium, 12, 56, 105, 187
Libritabs, 187
Lifestyle adjustment and education necessary to minimize bipolar disorder effects, 88–90
Light therapy as treatment for depression, 60, 75–76, 78, 156–157
Light-headedness and antipsychotic medications, 126
Limbic systems
    and anxiety, 104
    functions of, 29–30, 77
Limitations in knowledge of brain functioning, 38–39, 115
Lithium, 73, 90–94, 114–115, 128, 133, 137, 140–141, 145–146, 232–235
    dosage, 90–94
    and pregnancy and breastfeeding, 145–146
    expectations from taking, 94–95
Lithobid, 92, 232
Lithonate, 92, 232
Lithotabs, 92, 232
Liver and effects of anticonvulsant medication on, 95, 98
Locus coeruleus and panic, 112
Long-term antidepressant treatment, 69–70, 72–73
Lopressor, 178
Lorazepam, 105–106, 236–238
Loxapine, 123, 238–240
Loxitane, 123, 238
Loxitane C, Loxitane IM, 238
Ludiomil, 65, 241
Luvox, 65, 222
Managed care, benefits of in treatment of psychiatric conditions, 23, 58
Management of medications
    steps involved, 43–46, 61, 70–71, 99
    and doctor-patient cooperation, 39, 43–44, 46–47, 57, 63, 66–67, 74, 87, 89, 92–93, 96, 98, 100, 126, 144, 147–149, 159

Mania
    diagnosis and core symptoms of,
        82–85, 87, 96
    drug dosage rates, 91–93
    and hypomania, differences be-
        tween 83
    need for education and lifestyle
        changes, 88–90
Manic depression. *See* Bipolar disor-
    der; Depression; Mania
Manic psychosis, 117–118
MAO inhibitors antidepressants
    and borderline personality disor-
        der, 137
    as effective on brain chemicals in
        treatment of depression,
        62–63, 65, 77–78
    and effects on pregnancy and
        breastfeeding, 146
    potential dangers of, 63, 71–72,
        146
    as preferred treatment of bipolar
        disorders, 98
    and social phobia disorder,
        110–111
Maprotiline, 65, 240–243
Media, negative press and psychiatric
    drug developments, 10–12, 15–17
Medical disorders associated with
    psychiatric disorders, 55–56, 86,
    102–103, 117, 120–121, 140
Medical history
    for accurate diagnosis, 55, 103
    necessary in drug treatment, 41,
        43–44, 66, 99, 103, 114, 134,
        149
Medical treatment. *See* Treatment
Medication management. *See* Manage-
    ment of medications
Melatonin, 159
Mellaril, 122, 290
Mental Health Association, 60
Mental health specialists, training of,
    20–21
Mesoridazine, 122, 243–246
Metabolism as a process of drug dis-
    tribution within body, 40, 42–43
Methamphetamine, 174
Methedrine, 63
Methyldopa, 56
Methylphenidate, 63, 246–248
Metoprolol, 178
Miltown, 12
Mirtazapine, 65, 248–250
Midazolam, 105
Misconceptions of psychiatric disor-
    ders and historical approaches to
    treatment, 25–27
Misdiagnosis
    case histories, 13–14, 74

necessity of medical and psychi-
    atric evaluation to avoid,
    13–14, 20
Moban, 123, 251
Molidone, 123, 251–253
Mood changes as key to accurate
    diagnosis of schizophrenia,
    118–119
Mood
    disorders, prevalence of in U.S.
        7–8, 38
    and stabilizing medication for,
        87, 90–91, 97–98
    swings, 78, 81, 136–137, 140–141
MRI (magnetic resonance imaging),
    27, 132
Multiple personality disorder, 117
Multiple sclerosis as a cause of psy-
    chosis, 121
Nadolol, 178
Nardil, 65, 270
National Institute of Mental Health
    (NIMH), 7–8, 50, 61
Nausea. *See* Stomach upsets
Navane, 123, 293
Nefazodone, 65, 253–255
Nerve cells
    effected by antidepressant medi-
        cation, 60–62, 64
    implicated in psychiatric disor-
        ders, 28–33, 59–60, 64
    and Lithium, 91
    See also Neurotransmitters
Neuroleptic medication. *See* Antipsy-
    chotic medication, 90
Neuroleptic malignant syndrome
    (NMS), 126
Neurological side effects of antipsy-
    chotic medication, 125–126
Neurology and early psychotic disor-
    der misconceptions, 25–26
Neurotransmitters, malfunctions of
    and aging, 149–150
    and antidepressant medication,
        61–63, 65, 77–78
    and antianxiety medication, 106
    and diet, 75
    and dopaminergic medications,
        130
    and psychiatric disorders, 31–34,
        55, 87–88, 94–95, 112, 121,
        130
    and serotonin, norepinephrine,
        dopamine levels, 106, 130,
        157–158, 160
    and sleep patterns, 155
    See also Brain
Nimodipine, 57
Nocturnal myoclonus, 127–130
Norepinephrine (NE)

antidepressant medication and positive effect on, 59–62, 64–67, 73, 78, 112–113
malfunction of and psychological disorders, 59, 87, 32–33, 87–88, 112, 114
Norlutate, 57
Norplant, 57
Norpramin, 65, 73, 203
Nortriptyline, 65, 72, 255–258
Obsessive-compulsive disorder (OCD)
and antidepressants, 67, 116
diagnosis, 115
psychotherapy for, 35–36, 116
and increase in serotonin, 156–160
as type of anxiety disorder, 102
Ogen, 57
Olanzapine, 123, 258–260
Orap, 123, 273
Organic psychosis, 117, 120–121
Oxazepam, 105, 261–263
Pamelor, 65, 256
Panic disorder
and alternative methods to increase serotonin, 157–160
and atypical depression, 13–14, 78
and bulimia, 135
diagnosis and treatment, 111–113, 139
as type of anxiety disorder, 102
See also Anxiety; Depression; Drugs
Paranoia and borderline personality disorder, 136
Parkinson's disease and psychosis, 121, 141
Parkinsonian medication side effects, 125–126
Parnate, 65, 295
Paroxetine, 65, 263–265
Paxipam, 224
Paxil, 64–67, 157, 263
Pemoline, 265–267
Permitil, 217
Perphenazine, 123, 268–270
Personality and cosmetic psychopharmacology, 24–25
PET (positron emission tomography) to track metabolic functioning within brain, 27–28, 35–36, 58–59, 115–116, 132
Pharmacists as source of drug-drug interaction information, 22, 37, 63, 159
Pharmacokinetics, defined, 40–43
Pharmacology defined, 38–39
Phenelzine, 65, 270–273
Phenylpropanolamine, 113

Phobias
characterizations of and treatment for, 109–110
as type of anxiety disorder, 102
Physical symptoms as masking mental symptoms in diagnoses of psychiatric disorders, 13, 20
Physiological and psychological responses to minor stressful situations, 102, 104
Pimozide, 123, 273–275
Pindolol, 178
Polysomnography, 130
Porphyria and psychosis, 120
Post-traumatic stress disorder (PTSD), 138–140
Prazepam, 105
Pregnancy and medication, 70–71, 97–98, 143–146
Premarin, 57
Premenstrual dysphoria, 77–78, 103
Prescriptions, medical specialists licensed to write, 19–22
Prevalence of psychiatric disorders, 7–8, 38
Primary care physician as referral source for psychological treatment, 19–20, 89
Progestasert, 57
Progesterone and depression, 57
Prolixin, 123, 217
Prolixin decanoate, enanthate, 217
Propranolol, 105, 108, 110, 141, 178
Propranolol hydrochloride, 56
ProSom, 105, 212
Protriptyline, 22, 275–278
Provera, 57
Prozac, 16–17, 64–67, 73, 157, 214
Pseudolphedrine, 113
Psychiatric medication treatment
and children, 132, 147
goals of, 14, 34
referrals for, 19
Psychiatrists, 20–21
as licensed to prescribe medications, 21–22, 89
as providing psychotherapy for depression, 60
and relationship with psychotherapist in treatment of bipolar disorders, 88–89
and treatment for children and adolescents, 147
See also Psychotherapy
Psychoanalysis, 26
Psychologists, 20–21, 60
Psychopharmacology, 21, 38
Psychotherapist. *See* Psychotherapy
Psychotherapy

in conjunction with psychiatric medications treatment as effective, 2, 14, 20–23, 52, 59–61, 88–89, 113, 114, 116, 153, 137–138, 160
family, 148
group
for post-traumatic stress disorder, 137–138
for social phobias, 111
success in treatment dependent on severity of disorder, 9–10, 21, 153
as successful treatment of obsessive-compulsive disorder, 35–36
and treatment choice, 153
Psychosis. *See* Psychotic disorders; Schizophenia
Psychotic depression, 78–79, 117–119
Psychotic disorders
and aggression, 140
organic causes of, 120–121
prevalence of in U.S., 7–8, 38
types, 78–79, 83, 107, 117–120
Publicity, negative, and impact on public opinion of psychiatric drugs, 11–12, 15–17
Quality of life, 72, 89, 82
Quazepam, 105, 278–280
Quetiapine, 122, 280–283
Rapid cycling, 85–86
Reactive sadness verses depression, 51
Receptors defined, 39
Recordation of bipolar disorder episodes as self–care measure, 89
Recreation drugs
as cause of depression, 56
as cause of mania, 86
and disclosure of use, 44, 103
and nerve cell functioning, 33
See also Addiction
Referrals for diagnosis and treatment of psychiatric disorders, 2, 19, 21–22, 58, 60, 89, 147–148
Relapse, prevention of, 69, 72–73, 89
Relaxation training as effective for panic, 113
Remeron, 64–65, 248
Reptilian brain defined, 28
Reserpine, 32, 56
Research, limitations in understanding bipolar disorders, 87–88, 91
Restless legs syndrome, 129–130
Restlessness
as symptom of panic, 111, 127
as symptom of mania, 83–84
Restoril, 105, 288
Reuptake defined, 64

Risperdal, 123, 283
Risperidone, 100, 123, 283–285
Ritalin, 15–16, 132–133, 246
Ritalin SR, 246
Rituals and obsessive-compulsive disorder, 115
Safety
of antidepressant medication, 23, 69–72
of minor antipsychotic medication, 127
and antianxiety medication, 106–107, 110
and medications for children and adolescents, 145, 147–149
and medications during pregnancy, 97–98, 143–146
and stimulants, 133–134
Schizophrenia
causes and treatment, 120–121
diagnosis of, 31, 117–119
discovery of effective medications for, 10, 23, 38, 118
and doctor-patient trust, 46
and Thorazine, 26
Schizophreniform disorder, 118
Seasonal affective disorder (SAD), 75–76
Seizures
and mania, 86–87
risk of in medication treatment for anorexia and bulimia, 135
Self esteem
and attention deficit disorder, 131, 136, 147
and depression, 52–53, 61, 76–77, 84
Selective serotonin reuptake inhibitors (SSRIs), 63–64, 67, 73, 77–78, 98, 111, 135, 140–141, 157
Serax, 105, 261
Serentil, 122, 243
Serlect (Sertindole), 123
Seroquel, 122, 280
Serotonergic antidepressant treatment for obsessive-compulsive disorder, 35–36
Serotonin
as implicated in psychiatric disorders, 15, 33, 59–62, 64, 67, 77, 87, 114–116
and nonmedical approaches to regulate level of, 156–160
and norepinephrine, imbalance in as characteristic of psychological emotional disorders, 114–116, 157–158, 160
Ser-Ap-Es, 56
Serpasil, 56
Sertraline, 65, 285–287
Serzone, 65, 253

Sexual activity and psychiatric disorders, 54, 83–84
Side effects
    and antianxiety medications, 107–108
    and antidepressant medications, 16, 61–62, 64–67, 69–75, 110–111, 132–133
    of antipsychotic medications, 90, 124–127
    bipolar disorder treatment, 91–98
    defined, 39
    and the elderly, 150
    and early drug development, 27, 64
    all medications as producing, 14, 17, 61, 70
    and pregnancy and breastfeeding, 70–71, 97–98, 145–146
    and medications for children, 16, 149, 132–133
    and need for consultation with doctor, 2, 39, 66, 92–93, 98
    See also Drugs; Safety
Shock therapy. *See* Electro-convulsive therapy, 79–80
Sinemet, 57
Sinequan, 65, 209
Situational anxiety
    treatment for, 104–107
    as type of anxiety disorder, 102
Skin and effect of anticonvulsants on, 94–95
Sleep disorders, primary, 129–130
    disturbances
        and psychiatric disorders, 33, 52, 54–55, 59, 68, 76–78, 84–85, 89, 106–107, 114, 130
        light therapy for, 76
        and melatonin, 159
        as worsening psychiatric disorders, 154
    enhancement measures, 89, 155–156
Sleep apnea, 129–130
Social alienation as symptom of schizophrenia, 119
Social phobia
    diagnosis and treatment, 110–111
    as type of anxiety disorder, 102
SPECT (single photon emission tomography), 27–28, 58–59
Speech impairment as symptom of mania, 83
Spending sprees and symptom of mania, 84
St. John's Wort, 74, 159–160
Standard antidepressants, 56, 62, 64–65, 71
Stelazine, 123, 303

Stigmatization associated with psychiatric disorders and drug treatment for, 8, 16, 19, 101–102, 104, 108, 133–134
Stimulants
    as addictive, 71, 109
    association with psychiatric disorders, 86, 113, 119
    and attention deficit disorder, 132
    avoidance of with MAO inhibitor antidepressants, 63
    safety of, 133–134
Stomach upsets, 93, 95–97, 111
Storage of medications, 45, 162
Stress as interfering with normal brain nerve cell functioning, 33, 55, 59–60, 87, 101–102, 104, 108
    See also Post-traumatic stress disorder
Suicide and suicidal ideation
    and anxiety, 102
    and bipolar disorder, 82
    and borderline personality disorder, 136
    depression as contributing to, 50, 52, 54, 72, 79
    and negative publicity on drugs, 10–11, 16–17, 32
Support
    family, 56, 90, 120, 148
    group, 111, 139–140
Surmontil, 65, 306
Symmetrel, 57, 123, 176
Symptoms
    of anxiety disorders, 101, 111–112, 114
    of attention deficit disorder, 131
    of borderline personality disorder, 136
    and chemical brain malfunctions, 29–30
    of dementia, 141
    of post-traumatic stress disorder, 138–139
    types of, 38
    of mild depression in dysthymia, 76–77
    of major depression
        core, 51–55, 61, 68, 84
        physiological, 51, 54–56, 84–85
    of mania, core, 83–85, 89
    of psychotic disorders 117, 119–120
Systematic desensitization as psychological treatment of phobia, 110
Syphilitic infection
    as cause of depression, 56
    and psychotic disorder misconceptions, 25–26

Tacrine, 141
Talaga, 61
Talk therapy. See Psychotherapy
Tardive dyskinesia and antipsychotic
    medication, 124–125, 127
Technology
    growth of and impact on knowl-
        edge of brain, 27–28, 58–59
    and improvements in limiting
        medication side effects, 23
Tegretol, Tegretol XR, 94–95, 184
Temazepam, 105, 287–289
Tenormin, 105, 178
Thioridazine, 122, 290–292
Thiothixene, 123, 292–295
Thorazine, 26–27, 122, 190
Thorazine spansule, 190
Thought patterns
    as disorganized, 3, 79, 117, 119,
        121, 137
    negative, and depression, 54,
        76–77, 84
Thyroid, 73
    and anxiety, 103
    effects of Lithium on, 93–94
    hormones and depression, 73
Tofranil, 65, 229
Tofranil PM, 229
Tranquilizers
    and negative publicity, 11–12, 15–17
    minor, antianxiety medication as,
        71, 74, 104–107, 109, 112–114
Tranxene, 105, 199
Tranxene SD, 199
Tranylcypromine, 65, 295–298
Trazodone, 65, 298–301
Treatment
    for aggression, 140–141
    for attention deficit disorder,
        132–134
    for bipolar disorder
        and difficulty in treating
            rapid cycling pattern,
            85–86
        medication, 88, 90–99
        necessity of education and
            lifestyle change, 88
    for borderline personality disor-
        der, 137
    and debate on psychotropic
        medications prescribed for
        children and adolescents, 145,
        147–148
    for dementia, 141–142
    for depression
        medical and non-medical,
            59–80, 153–160
        ineffective, 74
    for generalized anxiety disorder,
        114–115

    for obsessive-compulsive disor-
        der, 116
    for panic disorder, 112–113
    for post-traumatic stress disorder,
        139–140
    for phobias, 109–111
    for situational anxiety, 104–106
    for schizophrenia, schizophreni-
        form, other psychotic disor-
        ders, 122–125
Treatment decisions
    factors to consider, 4
    and family, 148
    misconceptions promoting nega-
        tive, 8
Tremors, 93, 96, 125
Triazolam, 105, 301–303
Tricyclic antidepressant medication,
    16, 63–64, 72, 77–78, 86, 98
Trifluoperazine, 123, 303–305
Trihexyphenidyl, 123, 176
Trilafon, 123, 268
Tumor
    adrenal, as a cause of anxiety,
        103
    and psychosis, 119–121
Trimipramine, 65, 306–308
Tryptophan, 74
Tyrocine, 74
Valium, 12, 56, 71, 99, 105, 206
Valproate, 90–91, 95–96, 140–141,
    308–311
Valproic acid, 95–96, 146
Valrelease, 206
Variable nature of bipolar disorder, 82
Vascular diseases and psychosis,
    120–121
Venlafaxine, 65, 311–314
Verapamil, 100
Versed, 105
Visken, 178
Vistaril, 105, 107–108, 177
Vitamins
    as alternative treatment, 158
    deficiency and psychosis, 120
Vivactil, 65, 276
Weight
    and anorexia and bulimia,
        134–135
    and depression, 52, 54
    effects of medication on, 65, 94,
        97, 126
Wellbutrin, 64–67, 73, 135, 179
Wellbutrin SR, 179
Withdrawal, 106–108, 120, 124
Xanax, 105, 166
Zeldox (Ziprasidone), 123
Zoloft, 65–67, 73, 285
Zolpidem, 105, 314–315
Zyprexa, 123, 258

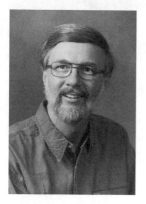

John Preston, Psy. D., is a clinical psychologist in private practice in Sacramento, California, and author of seven other books, including *You Can Beat Depression* and *Growing Beyond Emotional Pain*. He has taught on the faculty of the University of California at Davis School of Medicine, and is currently the chairman of the faculty for the Professional School of Psychology in Sacramento, California.

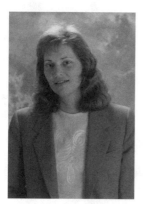

Mary C. Talaga, R.Ph., M.A., is Assistant Chief Pharmacist and Drug Education Coordinator for Kaiser Psychiatric Center, Sacramento, California. She has been a pharmacist for twenty years, specializing in psychiatric pharmacy for the last ten years. Ms. Talaga frequently gives in-service training on psychopharmacology and general pharmacy for school counselors and health care professionals.

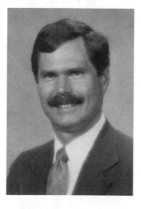

John H. O'Neal, M.D. has been a board-certified psychiatrist in private practice since 1977. A past chief of the Department of Psychiatry at Sutter Community Hospital in Sacramento, Dr. O'Neal is currently on the hospital staff. He is also an associate clinical professor of psychiatry at the University of California at Davis School of Medicine. He lectures on depression and psychopharmacology to mental health professionals, employee assistance programs, and the public. Dr. O'Neal received his M.A. in psychology from Harvard University.

Some Other New Harbinger Self-Help Titles